The Whitaker Wellness

Weight Loss Program

BY JULIAN WHITAKER, M.D.

Rutledge Hill Press®

Nashville, Tennessee

A Division of Thomas Nelson Publishers

www.ThomasNelson.com

To Julian, Conrad, Louisa, and Max Whitaker
Tammy, Angelina, David, and Shahana Faridi
Bret, Brandon, and Benjamin Boyd

Published by Rutledge Hill Press, a Division of Thomas Nelson, Inc., P.O. Box 141000, Nashville, Tennessee 37214.

Rutledge Hill Press books may be purchased in bulk for educational, business, fund-raising, or sales promotional use. For information, please e-mail SpecialMarkets@ThomasNelson.com.

Library of Congress Cataloging-in-Publication Data

Whitaker, Julian M.
    The Whitaker wellness weight loss program / by Julian Whitaker
    p. cm.
    Includes bibliographical references and index.
    ISBN 1-4016-0297-5 (hardcover)
    1. Reducing diets. 2. Weight loss. I. Title: Wellness weight loss program. II. Title.
    RM222.2.W43 206
    613.2'5—dc22

2005037512

Printed in the United States of America

06 07 08 09 10 — 5 4 3 2 1

CONTENTS

PREFACE

The twentieth century saw great advancements in sanitation, control of infectious diseases, childbirth, and trauma care that translated into an unprecedented increase in average lifespan. Today, however, we are facing a health challenge that threatens to reverse this upward trend: our growing epidemic of obesity.

In an insightful article entitled "A Potential Decline in Life Expectancy in the 21st Century," published in 2005 in the *New England Journal of Medicine,* leading aging researchers predicted dire consequences of this epidemic. "Looking out the window, we see a threatening storm—obesity—that will, if unchecked, have a negative effect on life expectancy. Despite widespread knowledge about how to reduce the severity of the problem, observed trends in obesity continue to worsen. These trends threaten to diminish the health and life expectancy of current and future generations."[1]

I have been practicing medicine for more than 30 years and have treated tens of thousands of patients at my clinic in Newport Beach, California, so I am well aware of the burden of diabetes, heart disease, cancer, and other consequences of obesity. However, I am unconvinced that there is "widespread knowledge about how to reduce the severity of the problem." If there were, we wouldn't have such a problem. Instead, there are scores of conflicting diet books and programs, each of them claiming to have the solution to obesity—and people looking for help are more confused than ever.

That's why I wrote the Whitaker Wellness Weight Loss Program. After researching and testing virtually every diet out there, I came to the obvious conclusion that the only way to achieve permanent weight control is to avoid foods that promote fat storage and discourage fat burning and return to the diet our bodies were designed to eat. It's high time this simple, scientifically proven, patient-tested concept, which has been buried under mountains of government-sponsored propaganda for decades, is recognized and put into practice. Only then will we stem the rising tide of obesity.

Like most projects, the Whitaker Wellness Weight Loss Program was a group effort. This book could not have been written without the superlative efforts of Peggy Dace, who has collaborated with me on many research, writing, and editing projects over the past 13 years. I would also like to thank Donna Sanford, Whitaker Wellness nutritionist, for her help with menu planning; Idel Kelly, Whitaker Wellness chef, for sharing her recipes; Sharon Barela and Madlen Simms for their research and contributions; Ryann Smith for her editing; and my wife Connie Whitaker for putting up with me. Additional thanks go to David McKenzie, who lit the fuse under this project, and Geoffrey Stone, our excellent editor at Rutledge Hill Press.

INTRODUCTION

If you've gone on diets in the past and lost weight only to regain it, you've picked up the right book. If you've had problems staying on any kind of weight loss regimen because of hunger and "lack of discipline," look no further. If you want to lose weight, lower your cholesterol and triglycerides, keep your blood sugar on an even keel, dramatically reduce your risk of diabetes and heart disease, and look and feel better than you have in years, then the Whitaker Wellness Weight Loss Program is for you.

What makes the Whitaker Wellness Weight Loss Program different from all the other diet books that promise similar results? It addresses the one thing that makes most weight loss programs fail: sticking with it. The average dieter loses his or her resolve in less than two months. Some people quit because they feel hungry all the time. Others get bored by limited food choices or give it all up for their favorite "forbidden" foods. More than a few get sidetracked and lose focus and discipline. Still others become discouraged because they don't see results fast enough.

What sets the Whitaker Wellness Weight Loss Program apart is that it provides you with all the tools you need to overcome hunger and food cravings, stay on track, and see results fast. How do I know? Because I've seen it work for my patients, who have no more or no less willpower or motivation than you.

The only thing you have to bring to the table to ensure success is a true desire to lose weight and an acceptance of the fact that this will require some changes in your life. If you are willing to make a commitment and follow this program, I guarantee that you will achieve your weight loss goals faster than you might anticipate—and keep weight off indefinitely.

Let's get started.

1

FINALLY, A DIET THAT REALLY WORKS

So you want to lose weight? Join the crowd. At any given time, at least half of all American adults are trying to do the same thing. That tells us a few things. First, we have an enormous weight problem in this country, and second, what we're doing about it just isn't working.

What we're not lacking are books and programs that promise to help you lose weight. This may surprise you, but I can tell you without hesitation that most weight loss diets do work, over the short term anyway—provided that you stick with them. But that's the problem. Most diets set you up for disappointment because they fail to address that most basic of human drives: hunger.

Hunger is a physiological need for food, a physical sensation that drives you to eat. It is controlled by an elaborate network of hormones, neurotransmitters, and other chemical messengers that tell you when to eat and when to stop. Hunger is a merciless taskmaster. Unfortunately, the typical weight loss diet is a prescription for hunger. Inadequate intake of calories or the wrong types of foods stimulate a series of biochemical reactions in the body that cause the brain to cry out, "Feed me!" When you cave in to these signals and eat, it's not because you are weak-willed or lacking in discipline. You are simply succumbing to an essential survival mechanism.

Another drawback of most weight loss programs is that they ignore the way the body stores and uses fat. Everybody knows we have an epidemic of obesity on our hands. Many experts blame it on large portion sizes—we just eat too much. There is some truth to this, but it's not as simple as eating less. Every bit as important as *how much* we're eating is *what* we're eating. Not all

1

foods affect the body the same way. Some foods, even when eaten in moderation, encourage fat deposition while others actually promote fat burning. If your food selections put you in the fat-storage mode, you can exercise all you want and you're still going to have trouble losing weight.

The good news is that you can control the hunger signals that are the bane of any dieter and rev up fat burning while decreasing fat storage. This, in a nutshell, is the foundation of the Whitaker Wellness Weight Loss Program. But before we delve into the details, let me tell you a little about the evolution of this program—and what it can do for you.

THE EVOLUTION OF THE WHITAKER WELLNESS WEIGHT LOSS PROGRAM

I've been practicing medicine in Orange County, California, since 1979, first in Huntington Beach and for the past 25 years in Newport Beach. It was only after I graduated from medical school that I discovered the healing power of nutrition and exercise—we certainly weren't taught such "frivolous" things in school—and it irrevocably changed the way I practice medicine. I wanted to help people get well, and I knew I couldn't do that within the confines of conventional medicine with its emphasis on drugs and invasive procedures.

I worked for a time at the Pritikin Institute, where I saw firsthand the tremendous therapeutic potential of diet and exercise. Not only did patients shed pounds, but they also shed diseases: heart disease, high blood pressure, diabetes, and other serious conditions. When I opened the Whitaker Wellness Institute shortly after that, I based it on the Pritikin model. Patients came for two weeks and stayed in a hotel near the clinic. Under my supervision, they exercised daily, ate a very low-fat diet, took nutritional supplements targeted at their specific health problems, and learned how to implement these lifestyle changes at home. My patients thrived on this program. They lost weight, discontinued drugs they'd been on for years, canceled surgeries, and truly got well.

There was one common criticism about the program, however: It was hard to stay on the diet after returning home. While many people adapted well, a good number of them complained of being hungry all the time and having a hard time keeping weight off over the long run. I couldn't understand it. Virtually all of America's leading health authorities and medical researchers were promoting a low-fat diet as the mecca of good health and weight control, plus I had filing cabinets full of supporting research. I truly believed that fat was the reason for all our ills from obesity to cancer to heart disease.

I was wrong. While some do very well on a low-fat diet, most people who struggle with weight do not. The reason is simple. If you aren't eating much fat or, by extension, much protein, you've got to be eating lots of something else, and that something else is carbohydrates. Even if you avoid sugars and white flour and eat only "healthy" brown rice; potatoes; and whole grain pasta, cereals, and breads, you are still subjecting yourself to a massive load of carbohydrates, and this, as I will explain in the next chapter, is working against your body's natural weight-control mechanisms.

Once I understood this concept, I began making changes in the Whitaker Wellness diet. I started using healthy fats such as olive oil more liberally. I added more protein from lean sources such as chicken and fish. And I cut back on starchy carbohydrates, offering only less carbohydrate-dense vegetables and fruits. And guess what? Patients loved it. They reported that it was easy to follow, and they lost more weight while continuing to reap all the health benefits of the stricter diet.

Over the years I've continued to make modifications in the diet, and the results just get better and better. In addition to following the latest scientific research, I've also depended on patient feedback to help shape this program. Nearly 40,000 patients have come to the Whitaker Wellness Institute over the past 27 years, and I've learned a lot from them: what works and what doesn't, what foods they like and dislike, and what changes they're willing or unwilling to make. In essence, the Whitaker Wellness Weight Loss diet is the culmination of almost three decades of in-the-trenches, hands-on patient experience.

In addition to the diet, this book also includes an exercise program. While you can lose weight on this dietary regimen even if you don't exercise, exercise makes it a heck of a lot easier. Furthermore, the health benefits of regular exercise are so profound that, as a physician, I would be remiss if I didn't do my best to encourage you to get active.

I've also included something that most programs lack: recommendations for specific foods and nutritional supplements that facilitate weight loss by reducing appetite or bumping up metabolism and increasing fat burning. Although, like exercise, they aren't critical for success, these supplements give many people a much-needed jump start on the track to weight loss.

Finally, I've included all of the tricks of the trade I've taught—and learned from—my patients over the years to help them commit to and stay with a weight loss program. One couple that can testify to the effectiveness of the Whitaker Wellness Weight Loss Program is Ken and Mourlene of Valley Springs, California.

Ken and Mourlene first came to my clinic in March of 2003. At that time Ken weighed 444 pounds. Prior to coming to Whitaker Wellness, they had tried to get Ken's weight under control without much success. Mourlene, who is French and a gourmet cook, realized that Ken's health was more important than the rich cuisine they both adored, and she had modified her recipes. But cutting back on fat didn't make much of a difference.

Obesity wasn't Ken's only problem. This 65-year-old also had diabetes, asthma, and chronic pain; and he was taking 12 prescription drugs. Recognizing that his weight was causing many of his health problems, we started Ken on the Whitaker Wellness Weight Loss diet, along with a comprehensive nutritional supplement regimen and additional therapies targeting his other health concerns. (Because Ken relied on a motorized scooter for mobility, exercise was out of the question initially.) Ken and Mourlene stayed in Newport Beach for two weeks while Ken underwent treatment. During that time, they ate meals prepared by our chef and, in lectures by our physicians and professional staff, learned about the causes of their health problems and how to implement solutions and lifestyle changes. At the end of their two-week stay, Ken had lost 25 pounds.

Mourlene wasn't in as bad of shape. She only had 20 to 30 extra pounds to conquer. After turning 50 and having a hysterectomy, Mourlene had gained almost 30 pounds. She made a pact with her husband to make a real change in their health, which is what prompted them to come to Whitaker Wellness.

They returned home with newfound knowledge and inspiration.

Mourlene realized that weight loss isn't all about reducing fat, and she quickly put the program into practice. For Ken, the improvements he experienced in that short period were just the carrot he needed. Two years later, Ken is a new man. He has lost 169 pounds and discontinued all of his medication. His blood sugar is under control—without drugs. He works out in the gym doing weight training a few times a week, walks a mile or two every day, and does yard and house work. (His scooter was gathering dust, so he sold it on eBay.) Ken now weighs 275 pounds and has no doubt he'll achieve his goal of losing 45 more.

Remarkable as Ken's story is, you may relate better to Mourlene's challenge: At her heaviest, Mourlene weighed 160 pounds. Today, she's down to an impressive 122, and she's kept the weight off. Mourlene stays on track with a daily routine of meditation, breathing exercises, and a workout with her bun and thigh roller. She also works in the yard almost every day and strives to stay active from 5:00 A.M. when she rises until she turns in for the night.

Mourlene and Ken's eating habits have changed dramatically. They eat lots of vegetables, some fruit, and moderate amounts of protein. They rarely eat out and often use protein shakes as meal replacements. Mourlene admits that one of the difficulties she encounters is entertaining dinner guests who still seem to expect the rich French dishes she used to prepare. But she and Ken don't miss them. "This program isn't a sacrifice; it's a part of our lives," she says.

WHAT'S IN STORE FOR YOU

Like Ken and Mourlene, you have a wonderful experience ahead of you. Let's jump ahead a month, six months, a year from now, after you're over the hump of changing old habits and this new lifestyle has become routine for you.

Envision the new you. You'll have shed unwanted pounds and taken inches off your waist and hips. You'll be wearing a smaller clothing size, and with your newly toned muscles, you'll look fabulous. And what you'll see in the mirror is only the tip of the iceberg. You'll feel different as well. You'll be invigorated and full of energy and vitality. You'll be sharper mentally, less anxious, and more upbeat. You'll be stronger and have more endurance. Even your sleep and sex life will improve!

I can promise all this and more because I've seen it time and again with patients at the Whitaker Wellness Institute. Just three weeks of focused attention on nutrition and exercise—the time it takes to break old habits and instill new ones—can set the stage for a lifetime of better health. That's because as important as the changes in how you look and feel are, more subtle changes are going on in your body. As you lose body fat, gain muscle, and feed your body the nutrients it thrives on, you'll be making dramatic improvements in virtually every aspect of your health.

INCREASED INSULIN SENSITIVITY

Extra weight, particularly if it's in the abdominal area, interferes with your body's ability to use insulin, a hormone we will be talking about a lot in this book. Insulin's job is to usher glucose, fat, and other nutrients into the cells. However, excess body fat causes the cells to lose their sensitivity to insulin's signals. The pancreas responds by releasing even more insulin, resulting in elevated levels of this hormone.

This is called insulin resistance, and it is linked not only with obesity but also with hypertension and abnormalities in cholesterol and triglycerides (fat in your blood). This cluster of conditions is so common that it has a name, metabolic syndrome (it's also called syndrome X), and it dramatically increases your risk of diabetes and heart attack. The Whitaker Wellness Weight Loss Program is as close to a sure cure for insulin resistance and metabolic syndrome as you can get, and as your cells become more sensitive to insulin's signals, you will reap a cascade of health benefits.

DECREASED RISK OF DIABETES

Type 2 diabetes is the end stage of insulin resistance—the cells become so insensitive to insulin that glucose cannot get in and blood sugar levels rise. We are currently experiencing an explosion of diabetes, and it is riding on the coattails of our epidemic of obesity. More than 80 percent of people with diabetes are overweight, and a gain of just 11 to 18 pounds doubles your risk of developing type 2 diabetes.

Weight loss is also a critical therapy for diabetes, and as your cells increase their sensitivity to insulin, all of the risk factors associated with diabetes will recede: heart attack and stroke, kidney disease, amputation, and blindness. Treating diabetes has been a specialty of mine for 30 years—I even wrote a book about it, *Reversing Diabetes*. My primary therapies are the diet and exercise program discussed in this book, along with targeted nutritional supplements.

LOWER CHOLESTEROL AND TRIGLYCERIDES

If your cholesterol and/or triglycerides are high, get ready to watch them fall on the Whitaker Wellness Weight Loss Program. One of my patients, Kerry, had exceptionally high blood lipids for years. When I first saw him, his triglycerides were 5,300 (normal is 100), his cholesterol was 490 (normal is less than 200), and his blood sugar was 590 (blood sugar of less than 100 is considered normal). Here is a guy who was headed for serious trouble. I told him to cut the sugar, bread, potatoes, and other starchy foods out of his diet, begin a walking program, and take fish oil capsules and other supplements.

After one month, his triglycerides fell to 764, his cholesterol to 260, and his blood sugar to 189. Three months later, his cholesterol was a respectable 186 and his triglycerides 303. And yes, Kerry achieved these remarkable improvements without Lipitor or any other prescription drug. These are the kinds of results you can expect on this program.

REDUCED BLOOD PRESSURE

High blood pressure and weight go hand in hand. The more body fat you have, the more blood vessels and capillaries you must have to nourish it—every extra pound or two of fat requires the addition of literally miles of extra blood vessels. This increases the resistance on the vessels and contributes to elevation of blood pressure.

A loss of just 10 percent of your current weight is often enough to lower blood pressure and provide tremendous health benefits.

DECREASED RISK OF HEART DISEASE

Lowering your cholesterol, triglycerides, blood pressure, and insulin resistance go a long ways toward guarding against heart disease. But as you lose weight, you'll gain even greater protection. A primary player in cardiovascular disease is inflammation. Most heart attacks occur when small plaques in the coronary arteries, destabilized by inflammation, rupture and attract a blood clot that blocks blood flow to the heart.

Where do these inflammatory compounds come from? In large part from your fat cells. Fat cells are not just a parking lot for excess calories but are metabolically active, churning out hormones and inflammatory chemicals. Excess body fat, especially in the abdomen, closely correlates with chronic inflammation. As this fat melts away, so do levels of harmful inflammatory compounds.

IMPROVEMENTS IN JOINT PAIN

If you're suffering with arthritis pain, weight loss will dramatically improve your symptoms. When you walk, your hips, knees, and ankles bear three to six times your total weight. This means that if you lose just 10 pounds, an additional 30 to 60 pounds of extra stress will be lifted off your joints.[1]

Even if you don't have arthritis, losing weight will decrease your risk of developing it in the future. This is because extra weight hastens the breakdown of cartilage. Obesity is the leading cause of arthritis in women and the second leading cause, after sports injuries, in men—it quadruples risk of arthritis of the knee in women and increases it five-fold in men. Even moderate weight loss decreases strain on weight-bearing joints, improves symptoms, and slows the progress of arthritis.[2]

PROTECTION AGAINST CANCER

Your risk of cancer will also fall, especially if you are extremely overweight. Experts estimate that excess weight accounts for up to 20 percent of all deaths from cancer. In a 16-year American Cancer Society study of more than 900,000 adults, extreme obesity increased the death rate from cancer by 52 percent in men and 62 percent in women.[3]

But even moderate weight gain may increase risk. That's because fat cells produce a number of hormones and other substances that may stimulate cancer growth. Maintaining normal weight has been shown to be protective against cancers of the breast, uterus, gallbladder, cervix, ovary, prostate, and colon.

LOWER RISK OF MAJOR DISEASES

As you lose weight, your likelihood of encountering many other health challenges will also diminish. One of them is nonalcoholic fatty liver disease, the leading liver problem in this country, which affects roughly one in four Americans. You'll also be less prone to developing gallstones and gallbladder disease, gout, sleep apnea, and perhaps even Alzheimer's disease. All in all, excess weight is one of our country's leading causes of premature, preventable death—second only to smoking.

In summary, when you combine the protective effects of weight reduction with the proven health-enhancing effects of the lifestyle changes in the Whitaker Wellness Weight Loss Program, you'll be on the road to excellent health.

2

INSTANT DISCIPLINE

No program, weight loss or otherwise, is going to work unless you follow it. This requires mustering the discipline to make changes in your behavior. Nobody likes to make changes. It's painful. That's why so many people fail at dieting, exercising, stopping smoking, or anything else that requires a change in behavior. Only if the pain of *not* changing outweighs the pain of changing will you succeed.

Let's take smoking as an example. (As Mark Twain said, "Quitting smoking is easy. I've done it thousands of times.") Say you're a smoker and you want to quit. Imagine that everywhere you go for three weeks a big guy with a baseball bat follows you around. You know that if you so much as take one puff of a cigarette, he will hit you hard in the back of the head. What are the chances of lighting up if you know you're going to get hit in the head with a bat?

In order to change any behavior you have to put a guy behind you with a baseball bat. You need to create a painful consequence for flaking out that hurts worse than the discomfort of not giving into the behavior you want to stop. It's that simple—instant discipline.

Since you most likely won't have someone at the ready to whomp you upside the head every time you eat a Krispy Kreme or fail to exercise, you need to come up with another disincentive that hits you where it really hurts: your wallet.

MY OWN STORY

A few years ago, I was fat. I'm often introduced as America's Wellness Doctor, but at that time I looked like the Pillsbury Doughboy. The cause of my corpulence was no mystery. I had lost the discipline and energy necessary to do what I knew I needed to do to control my weight, and the result was embarrassing. Therefore, I made a commitment to lose 20 pounds in two and a half months. Ten weeks, two pounds a week—it was definitely doable. To hold myself accountable I did two things.

First, I boldly declared my goal in my monthly newsletter, *Health & Healing*. As it goes out to hundreds of thousands of subscribers, mine was quite a public pronouncement. Furthermore, I promised to let readers know how I did in a future issue, so there would be no conveniently ignoring the issue if I failed in my weight loss goal.

Second, I made a bet, a written contract that I dated, signed, had witnessed, and posted in a prominent place. I bet that either I'd lose the 20 pounds in two and a half months or I would send $10,000 to my least favorite charity. To make a long story short, I succeeded. Here's how I did it.

I do not have extraordinary willpower. In fact, I've lost and regained weight more times than I care to admit. One thing that kept me on track in this particular instance was my public declaration. The specter of humiliation is a powerful motivator. Everybody around me knew I was trying to lose weight. My family, my staff, patients at the clinic, everybody seemed to know about my weight loss goal and would frequently ask me how it was going. I also knew I was going to have to print the results, and the thought of admitting to several hundred thousand people that I failed was much more painful than putting on my running shoes and hitting the road.

The other thing that motivated me was my wager—it stiffened my resolve like quick-set concrete. I don't make bets lightly. I was fully prepared to write out a check to my least favorite charity in the event that I came up short. But donating such a large sum of money to a cause that was so odious to me was, like the thought of public humiliation, far, far more agonizing than passing on crème brûlée and chocolate cake.

PERSONAL ACCOUNTABILITY

The reason this method works so well is because it increases your personal accountability. Accountability is simply your responsibility to someone or for some action. In essence, it's no more than character. You say you're going to do something, so you do it. You run into accountability in every aspect of your life. You're accountable to your boss for doing your job in a timely and acceptable manner. You're accountable to your spouse for meeting the needs that only a husband or wife can meet, and to your kids for providing a safe, nurturing, and loving environment. You're accountable to your friends for showing up at scheduled get-togethers and to the government for paying your taxes.

In every one of these cases you choose to take responsibility, and there are significant consequences if you fail. If you don't do what is expected of you at work, you'll get fired. If you repeatedly let your family down, you'll likely end up in divorce court. If you stand your friends up, you'll eventually lose them. If you don't pay taxes, you'll go to jail.

Yet personal accountability is a horse of a different color. If your actions or lack thereof affect only yourself, it's a lot easier to act irresponsibly, and this is particularly true of health habits. If I hadn't lost those 20 pounds, I wouldn't have lost my job, and my wife wouldn't have left me. If I had not made my goal public, the only one I would have let down was myself. Nobody would have known that I had planned to give up pasta, and I could have easily convinced myself to start exercising "tomorrow."

So when you're really ready to lose weight, increase the consequences of failure. Go public with your plans so you'll risk losing face. Let humiliation motivate you. Make a bet to do something you really, really don't want to do, payable only if you skirt personal responsibility. Pledge a sum of money to a cause or individual that is completely out of sync with your values, and make it large enough that it'll hurt if you have to cough it up. Because most of us have no trouble breaking promises to ourselves, let's up the ante. I tell you, it works.

PLEDGE TO CHANGE YOUR BEHAVIOR

I've made one significant modification to this motivation technique over the years. My pronouncement that I was going to lose 20 pounds in two and a half months wasn't very smart because it wasn't something that I had total control over. True, it was a reasonable goal for me, but it left me wide open for failure. Even though I did everything right during that time period and inevitably lost weight, I still might have fallen short of the 20-pound mark. If I'd lost 17 or 18 pounds, I should have been ecstatic; instead, I would have been writing a check I really didn't want to write. I was sweating bullets the entire two and a half months, but I ended up coasting across the finish line with a loss of 24 pounds.

What I learned from this experience is the importance of pledging to change your *behavior*, rather than vowing to lose a specific number of pounds. Of course, you'll likely be aiming at a target weight, but if you focus on your behavior—what you eat and how much you exercise—weight loss will naturally follow. Your behavior is the only thing that's 100 percent under your control.

Another thing I learned is that it's better to make your commitments in smaller chunks of time. Don't say you're going to exercise every day for the rest of your life. Start out with five days a week for several weeks—with the intention of renewing your commitment. I would suggest starting with three weeks. Conventional wisdom says it takes three weeks to break a habit, and even if that's not true, it's a reasonable period of time: long enough to challenge you yet short enough to see the end in sight.

So get your calendar out and sit down with a pen and paper. It's not enough to want to lose weight. You've got to make a plan. Decide on the behaviors you're willing to change and the day you want to start. Think about the most loathsome cause or individual you would have to reward in case you break your contract, and pledge to donate a significant sum to that entity if you break your promise. Do not pledge a trifling sum; make it count. For some it might be $25; for others, $2,500.

Be very specific. After you become familiar with the particulars of the Whitaker Wellness Weight Loss Program, you may be ready to embrace the whole enchilada. (Chapter 14 includes a three-week meal plan, and Chapter 10 outlines a specific exercise program.) If you're unwilling to go full throttle, then select aspects of the program that you are willing to do. Perhaps you're ready to get serious about exercise, or you're willing to commit to just one segment of the diet such as giving up bread and other starches. Think this through carefully, because you are about to make a solemn promise to a very important person: yourself. Then write it down in a format similar to the contract below, sign and date it, and have it witnessed.

COMMITMENT CONTRACT

I,_____ agree to _____

for three weeks beginning _____. If I so much as

_____

I agree to give $_____ to _____

Signed _____

Witnessed by _____ Date _____

I've seen a lot of contracts over the years. Mike, an avid hunter, pledged, "I agree to stop eating desserts for three weeks. If I so much as eat one dessert, I agree to give $1,000 to PETA." (PETA is an animal rights organization that opposes hunting.) Here's what Charlie, a staunch Republican, came up with: "I agree to stop smoking for three weeks. If I so much as take one puff, I agree to give $100 to the Democratic National Party." Raquel, a Diet Coke junkie and shopaholic, turned the pain of failing into a reward for succeeding: "I agree to stop drinking Diet Coke for three weeks. If I drink no Cokes for three weeks, I will treat myself to a $200 shopping spree."

The next step is to broadcast your pledge to everybody you know: family, friends, coworkers, anybody who will listen. Make sure they know what you're doing and the consequences of failure. If someone at work offers you a doughnut, tell them why you're turning it down. If a friend wants to meet you at a time you've previously scheduled for exercise, explain why you'll have to put it off an hour. Most of the people in your life will support and encourage you. A few may attempt to thwart you. But make no mistake. Friends and enemies alike will know if you fall off the wagon.

I have helped hundreds of patients over the years improve their health with this technique. I can always tell if someone really wants to make the changes they claim they want to make. Those who are truly serious make a contract. Those who aren't make excuses. Regardless of how much lip service people may give, if they won't sign a contract, they know they won't make the effort to change.

No matter what personal health behavior you want to modify—stopping smoking, drinking less, cutting out problem foods such as candy bars or sodas, exercising regularly—this method works. And when the behavior is controlled, results automatically follow.

THE PLEASURE-PAIN PRINCIPLE

Okay, you've made a commitment, selected the specific behaviors you're planning to change, and signed your contract. If you've taken this as seriously as I hope you have, the hardest part is over. Now all you have to do is stay focused for the next 21 days. Throughout this book I provide tips for helping you stay on track. I've devoted an entire chapter to exercise, and it's full of practical suggestions. The diet is specifically designed to sidestep the primary stumbling block of most other weight loss programs—you won't be hungry all the time. In addition, there are chapters dedicated to helping you curb your appetite and burn more fat. All told, these will help you stay on the straight and narrow. But nothing is more powerful than your contract with yourself.

I'm not going to sit here and tell you it will be a piece of cake (pardon the expression). There will be moments when you'll have to wrestle with temptation. If you're like me and most of my patients, your biggest challenge may be giving up bread, snack foods, desserts, and other starchy, sugary foods that have become such a dominant part of the typical American diet. Here's how you lick it.

It's called the pleasure-pain principle. Let's say you're at lunch, and everyone around you is eating pizza. A piece of thick-crust pizza has some positive aspects, no doubt about it. It looks good, it smells good, and since your friends are enjoying it so much, you know it tastes good. You have a positive, pleasurable stimulus to eating that pizza. But there is also a negative stimulus: It's a breach of your contract. One bite of pizza and you're sending out a check to your least favorite individual or organization.

If you're dining with friends, everyone at that table knows about your contract and that if you eat that pizza, you're going to have to cough up a sizeable donation to your least favorite charity. Make the pain far more significant than the pleasure, and you have built-in discipline, the strength of which will astound you. If the road to hell is paved with good intentions, then the road to heaven is paved with executed contracts.

TRACKING YOUR SUCCESS

Once you get started, you're going to be looking for results, and one of the best things about the Whitaker Wellness Weight Loss Program is you will see results quickly. I encourage you to track your accomplishments, but realize there are several ways to measure success, and they don't all involve stepping on a bathroom scale.

First and foremost, make your health behaviors your primary focus. If you are eating right and exercising, you will lose weight. (Actually, you'll lose weight on this program even if you don't exercise, but exercise will speed it up and make it easier to maintain—in addition to numerous other health benefits.) I cannot predict exactly how much you'll lose each week because everyone is different. While most of you will start shedding pounds the very first week, weight loss may be more gradual for some. But I promise that if you change your behavior, results will follow.

Second, be realistic when setting your weight loss goals. Recognize that our culture showcases unrealistic, rigid, and often unattainable ideals of beauty that are out of sync with the average healthy physique. I know I can't convince you of this in a paragraph, but you don't have to be fashion-model thin to be healthy and happy with your weight. Genetically, it's not in the cards for most people. I would like to look like Arnold Schwarzenegger did 20 years ago—I'm sure Arnold Schwarzenegger would like to look like he did 20 years ago—but it's not going to happen. Accept what you've got to work with, learn to love your body type, and don't torment yourself trying to be something you're not. (See Chapter 4 for more on genetics and body type.)

Next, decide on a tracking system that works for you. For most, it will probably be regular weigh-ins. I could give you a number of formulas for determining your ideal weight. Body mass index (BMI) is used by most physicians and research scientists to calculate obesity, and while it is a useful tool, it's not 100 percent accurate. Athletes and other individuals with a lot of muscle mass may have BMIs suggesting they are obese, even if they have no excess body fat. On the other hand, a sedentary individual with little muscle mass and more body fat may have a "normal" BMI. Decide on a *realistic* weight and aim for it.

Another way to track your progress is by measuring the circumference of your waist and hips. This is also used in medicine to determine obesity and, in fact, the waist-to-hip ratio is now considered to be a better marker of health than BMI. That's because, as we discussed in the first chapter, weight carried in the abdominal area is a greater health hazard than extra pounds in the thighs or buttocks. Ratios aside, waist and hip circumferences are a pretty good way of monitoring fat loss, which is what you're really after. If you are doing resistance exercises, you're gaining muscle as well as losing fat. Because muscle tissue weighs more than fat, you may not be losing pounds as fast as you'd like, but you are improving your body composition (more muscle, less fat), and this will make permanent weight control much easier.

To determine your waist circumference, take a measuring tape and measure your bare waist at its narrowest point. For men, this will be right at the navel, and for women, about an inch below the navel. To measure your hips, men should aim for the tip of the hipbones and women for the widest area between the hips and buttocks. The tape measure should be taut but not pulled so tight that it compresses the skin. Jot your numbers down and record weekly.

Or you can dispense with these things altogether. One of the best ways of tracking weight loss is by looking in the mirror. How do you look? How do your clothes fit? That's what Elizabeth did. When I first saw her, Elizabeth was dressed in a loose-fitting shirt and slacks. She said she always wore sweats and baggy tops to cover up her body, which strained a size 12. She embraced the program wholeheartedly and particularly concentrated on exercise: skiing, ice skating with her children, and playing tennis three or four times a week. I saw her ten weeks later. Although she had only lost six pounds, she was amazed that she had lost eight inches and dropped two dress sizes, down to an 8—and she looked stunning in a suit with a short black skirt. The lesson here is, don't be a slave to the scale—measure your progress by how you look and feel.

PUTTING IT ALL TOGETHER

Let's return to the title of this chapter, "Instant Discipline." The bugaboo of every weight loss plan is compliance. Recognizing that you're overweight, realizing the health problems associated with obesity, wanting to lose weight, even knowing how to go about it: None of these is enough to make you stick with the pain of giving up favorite foods and exercising regularly. As I've said, if you're going to manage to make permanent changes in your behavior, you're going to have to up the ante and make the pain of not doing the things required to lose weight more compelling than the pleasure of doing them.

In summary, you need to make a commitment to change a specific behavior. Decide on a pleasure-pain incentive that really means something—make failure hurt—and put it in writing, along with a starting and ending date. Tell everyone you know about your pledge and enlist their support in helping you stay on track. Then just do it. I can't tell you how proud you will be of yourself in three weeks, once you've proved to yourself that you can do this . . . in three months, when you and everyone around you can see how great you look . . . and in three years, when a good diet and regular exercise have long since become a normal part of your life.

That's exactly what happened with Franceen as she explained in the following letter:

When I first came to the Whitaker Wellness Institute I was not well. I had high blood pressure, triglycerides, cholesterol, and blood sugar, not to mention I was overweight. My emotional health was very poor as well. My hormones were off-balance and I was feeling very discouraged.

My doctor set me up on a wonderful, life-changing program of herbs and vitamins as well as a diet to help me control my medical problems, eating habits and lose weight. Everyone at the Institute—from the doctors to the nurses to the nutritionist—gave me instructions, assistance, and encouragement throughout, and I left with a clear plan for regaining my health.

Now six months later I have the physical and emotional control I was searching for. My blood pressure, triglycerides, cholesterol, and blood sugar levels are all normal. My hormones are balanced, and my eating habits are finally under control. I have a new lifestyle! I have lost 18 pounds and I am still losing. I went from a dress size 16 to a size 10. I exercise daily and have never felt better. Thanks to all!

GET INTERACTIVE

Let us help you lose weight. At www.whitakerweightloss.com, you'll find additional tools for getting started and staying on the Whitaker Wellness Weight Loss Program. You'll be able to print out commitment contracts and exercise logs. You'll find additional recipes and advice on eating out, exercising, and keeping on track. You can also sign up for e-mail reminders, words of encouragement, and other tips for honoring your commitment. I encourage you to visit our website. It's just one more way we can help you instill the habits that will result in permanent weight loss and a lifetime of better health.

Visit www.whitakerweightloss.com to get started.

3

WHY WE'RE FAT

You know the statistics. Sixty-five percent of American adults and 15 percent of our kids are overweight, and 30 percent of us—60 million people— are obese.[1] There is no shortage of explanations for why we have weight problems and, believe me, I've heard them all. "Everybody in my family is fat." "I don't eat that much but I still put on weight." "Most everyone gains weight after 50." "My metabolism is too slow." "It's my hormones." "I'm unable to exercise." "This drug I'm taking has made me balloon up."

All of these things do contribute to weight gain, and when I sit down with a patient to work on weight issues, we certainly factor them in. However, none of them can explain the unprecedented epidemic of obesity that has swept across America in the past 25 years. According to the Centers for Disease Control, the number of obese adults doubled from 1980 to 2000, and the number of overweight children has tripled.[2]

The enormity of this increase is particularly striking when you consider how fast it has come on. Only in the past 50 years has obesity been an issue at all. Of course, there have always been heavy people, but they were the exception, not the rule. During the 1960s and 1970s, obesity rates were generally level, hovering around 14 percent. Approximately 45 percent of adults were overweight, and only 5 percent of our kids had a weight problem.[3]

The early 1980s, however, saw the beginning of an upward trend that has continued unabated ever since. During that time, the number of overweight adults increased by 20 percentage points—almost 1 percent per year! Twenty years ago, type 2 diabetes, which is endemic in overweight adults, was virtually unheard of in children; but now that one in six kids is overweight, it is showing up in record numbers. Even the nomenclature has been blurred. Because children are now developing type 2 diabetes, no longer is type 1 diabetes referred to as juvenile diabetes, nor can type 2 be called adult-onset diabetes. From larger, sturdier furniture and resized clothing to seatbelt extenders and bigger coffins, the fattening of America cannot be ignored.

What happened? What has occurred in the past 25 years that could possibly explain this phenomenon?[4]

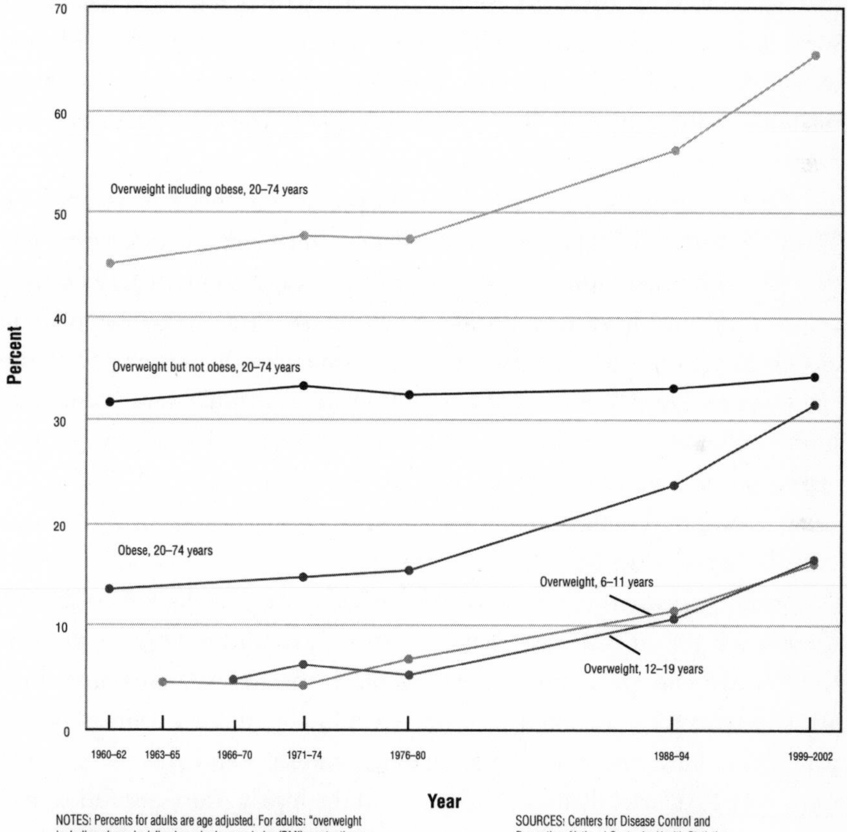

Figure 16. Overweight and obesity by age: United States, 1960–2002

NOTES: Percents for adults are age adjusted. For adults: "overweight including obese: is defined as a body mass index (BMI) greater than or equal to 25, "overweight but not obese" as a BMI greater than 25 but less that 30, and "obese" as a BMI greater than or equal to 30. For children: "overweight" is defined as a BMI at or above the sex- and age-specific 95th percentile BMI cut points from the 2000 CDC Growth Charts: United States. "Obese" is not defined for children. See Data Table for data points graphed, standard errors, and additional notes. Data are for the civilian noninstitutionalized population and are age adjusted. See Data Table for data points graphed and additional notes.

SOURCES: Centers for Disease Control and Prevention, National Center for Health Statistics, National Health Examination Survey and National Health and Nutrition Examination Survey.

Centers for Disease Control and Prevention, National Center for Health Statistics. Health, United States, 2004

CAVEMAN GENES, MODERN WORLD

We can debate this question until we're blue in the face, but when you step back and look at the big picture, there is only one logical answer: America's obesity epidemic is caused by our dramatically increased consumption of starches and sugars over the past 25 years.

Let's start by looking at it from an evolutionary perspective. What is the human body designed to eat? One expert in this field, S. Boyd Eaton, M.D., popularized the concept of the Paleolithic diet in the 1980s and claimed that our hunter-gatherer ancestors ate mostly fruits and vegetables with some lean meat. Their diet was low in fat, especially saturated fat, with lots of high-fiber carbohydrates and only moderate amounts of protein. Others, including Loren Cordain, Ph.D., author of *The Paleo Diet*, believe that the caveman diet was much higher in fat and protein.

We may never know exactly what our prehistoric ancestors ate, but it's easy to go back in history and figure out what they *didn't* eat. We know that for most of human evolution, they did not eat cereal grains or refined sugars, nor did they have access to dairy products, refined vegetable oils, or alcohol. That's because agriculture didn't come onto the scene until about 10,000 years ago. The advent of agriculture was a seminal development in human civilization. As people moved away from nomadic groups into larger, stable communities, cultural advancements exploded. But other changes occurred as they took up farming and domesticated livestock, and one of them was the basic human diet.

You may be thinking, so what? We've been eating bread and sugar and the like for 10,000 years, and our lifespan is at an all-time high. Consider this. Based on archaeological evidence available to date, experts estimate that 100,000 generations of *Homo sapiens* were hunter-gatherers, while only 500 generations have lived since the dawn of agriculture—and only two generations have had virtually unlimited access to the highly processed foods that are a mainstay of the American diet. Ten thousand years is the blink of an eye in terms of evolution. We may be living in the modern world, enjoying the snacks, takeout meals, and convenience foods that technology has made possible, but we still have caveman genes.

The problem, according to a 2005 article by Dr. Cordain, Dr. Eaton, and others in the *American Journal of Clinical Nutrition*, is "the collision of our ancient genome with the new conditions of life in affluent nations, including the nutritional qualities of recently introduced foods." The article continues: "There is growing awareness that the profound environmental changes (e.g., in diet and other lifestyle conditions) that began with the introduction of agriculture and animal husbandry approximately 10,000 years ago occurred too recently on an evolutionary time scale for the human genome to adapt. In conjunction with this discordance between our ancient, genetically determined biology and the nutritional, cultural, and activity patterns in contemporary Western populations, many of the so-called diseases of civilization have emerged."[5]

And at the top of that list, casting a dark shadow over virtually every system in the body, is obesity.

CARB CRAZY

Of all the post-Paleolithic foods, none occupies a larger place on our plates than sugars and starches. Our per capita sugar consumption is off the charts at 152 pounds per year, up 30 pounds since 1970. Even more ominous are starches. More than 85 percent of the grains eaten in the U.S. diet are refined and highly processed. Although none of you can be lulled into thinking that Snickers and Twinkies are good for you, we've been brainwashed over the past 25 years into believing that most other carbohydrates are man's best friend.

Gary Taubes, in an eye-opening article in the respected scientific journal, *Science*, says that America's carb craze dates back to 1977, when a U.S. Senate committee issued a report entitled "Dietary Goals for the United States," urging Americans to eat less fat. This report, which was based on rather sketchy scientific evidence, maintained that fat raised cholesterol levels and was thus a primary cause of heart disease. Therefore, the cure for our country's ills was determined to be reducing fat in the diet. Hundreds of millions of dollars were spent on research trying to solidify the link between dietary fat and heart disease. Despite the fact that not a single study was able to validate this theory, the die was cast, and the low-fat phenomenon developed a life of its own.[6]

Virtually every public health agency and health authority—myself included—bought into it. We truly believed that the path to wellness was paved with low fat. Of course, something had to replace fat in the diet. Protein was suspect because most protein-dense foods such as meat and eggs also contain fat. Therefore, through a process of elimination, the onus fell on carbohydrates.

Somewhere along the line, carbohydrates were also crowned the ideal foods for weight loss. The reasoning went that because a gram of fat contains nine calories while a gram of carbohydrate contains only four, then less fat and more carbs translated into eating fewer calories. Little did we realize, as I will explain below, that the result of this 25-year experiment would be a dramatic increase in calories, accompanied by inevitable weight gain.

The pinnacle of the high-carbohydrate movement came in 1992 with the release of the Food Guide Pyramid from the U.S. Department of Agriculture (USDA), which replaced the four food groups that had been around for 35 years. I attended grade school in Atlanta in the 1950s, and I clearly remember the posters in our classrooms depicting the "Basic Four": milk, meat, fruits and vegetables, and breads and cereals. What I didn't know at the time was that the food industry played a major role in putting these recommendations together. (The National Dairy Council was responsible for placing those posters in schools.) Nor did I realize when I accepted the low-fat dogma back in the seventies that industry insiders also wielded considerable influence on the creation of the food pyramid.[7]

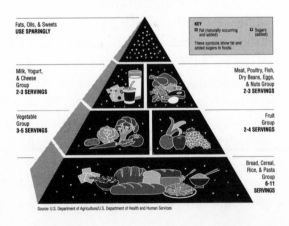

Food Guide Pyramid
A Guide to Daily Food Choices

Fats, Oils, & Sweets
USE SPARINGLY

KEY
◻ Fat (naturally occurring and added)   ◻ Sugars (added)
These symbols show fat and added sugars in foods.

Milk, Yogurt, & Cheese Group
2-3 SERVINGS

Meat, Poultry, Fish, Dry Beans, Eggs, & Nuts Group
2-3 SERVINGS

Vegetable Group
3-5 SERVINGS

Fruit Group
2-4 SERVINGS

Bread, Cereal, Rice, & Pasta Group
6-11 SERVINGS

Source: U.S. Department of Agriculture/U.S. Department of Health and Human Services

The food pyramid had an enormous impact on our eating habits. At its base was a recommendation to eat 6 to 11 servings per day from the bread, cereal, rice, and pasta group, and at its pinnacle an admonition to use fats and oils sparingly. Manufacturers took this and ran with it, creating entire lines of low-fat and fat-free food. Cookies, candy, cake, margarine, cheese, you name it: If a label boasted reduced fat or no cholesterol, consumers would buy it. Never mind that the fat in these products was replaced by starches and sugars. "Nonfat" was considered to be synonymous with health. By the time the mid-1990s rolled around, almost three-quarters of American shoppers considered fat content in making food purchases.

Between 1971 and 2000, the average number of calories consumed by Americans increased from 2,450 to 2,618 for men and 1,542 to 1,877 for women. Virtually all of this 168 to 335 calorie increase came in the form of carbohydrates. Carbohydrates as a percentage of total caloric intake rose by approximately 6.5 percentage points, contributing about 65 extra grams of carbohydrate per day. Meanwhile, fat consumption decreased by about 4 percentage points, and there was also a slight decrease in calories from protein.[8]

FIGURE 1: Percentage of kilocalories from macronutrient intake among men aged 20–74 years*, by survey years—National Health and Nutrition Examination Surveys (NHANES), United States, 1971–2000

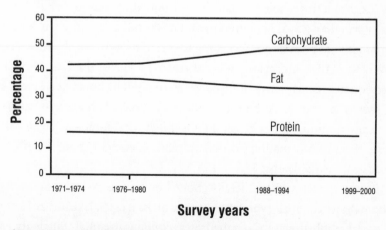

Survey years

*Age adjusted by direct standardization to the 2000 U.S. Census population by using age groups 20–39, 40–59, and 60–74 years.

FIGURE 2: Percentage of kilocalories from macronutrient intake among women aged 20–74 years*, by survey years—National Health and Nutrition Examination Surveys (NHANES), United States, 1971–2000

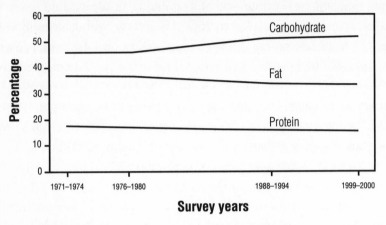

*Age adjusted by direct standardization to the 2000 U.S. Census population by using age groups 20–39, 40–59, and 60–74 years.

Yet contrary to government expectations, Americans continued to get fatter and fatter. High cholesterol levels and hypertension are still major problems, and while heart disease rates have abated somewhat over the past 20 years, nothing suggests that it's because we've been eating less fat. At the same time, rates of diabetes and other diseases linked to obesity are soaring.

Turns out, this whole low-fat high-carbohydrate nonsense has done far more harm than good. That food pyramid was officially retired in 2005, but the damage has been done. According to one of its most vocal critics, Walter C. Willett, M.D., professor and chairman of Harvard's Department of Nutrition, its departure was long overdue. In his 2001 book, *Eat, Drink, and Be Healthy,* he wrote, "At best, the USDA pyramid offers wishy-washy, scientifically unfounded advice on an absolutely vital topic—what to eat. At worst, the misinformation contributes to overweight, poor health, and unnecessary early deaths."[9]

Before we get into the details about how eating excessive amounts of carbohydrates can make you fat, I want to make it crystal clear that I am not bashing carbohydrates. Carbohydrates contain essential nutrients, and many of our most healthful foods such as vegetables and fruits are composed primarily of carbohydrates. You can eat vegetables to your heart's content, along with moderate amounts of fruit, and never, I mean *never,* have a weight problem.

But the bulk of the carbohydrates we eat are not vegetables and fruits. Although half of the average American's calories come from carbs, I guarantee that people are not filling up on broccoli and blueberries. Fewer than one in four adults eats the recommended five-plus servings of vegetables and fruits a day. The carbohydrates that fill our plates are not found in the produce aisle but in the packaged and frozen foods that take up most of your supermarket shelf space. As Gary Taubes points out in the article I cited earlier, "The food industry has little incentive to advertise nonproprietary items: broccoli, for instance. Instead . . . the great bulk of the $30-billion-plus spent yearly on food advertising goes to selling carbohydrates in the guise of fast food, sodas, snacks, and candy bars. And carbohydrates are all too often what Americans eat."[10]

Even if you eschew junk food and eat only "healthy" carbohydrates such as pasta, whole grain bread, orange juice, and sugar-free breakfast cereals, you may still have trouble losing pounds or maintaining your ideal weight. That's because all carbohydrates, to one degree or another, stimulate the release of insulin. Insulin is a powerful hormone that affects both appetite and fat storage. And that, my friend, is the crux of the carbohydrate conundrum.

THE CARBOHYDRATE CONUNDRUM

Carbohydrates come in various forms, from one- or two-sugar molecules such as fructose (found in fruits) and lactose (milk sugar) to long chains of glucose linked together (starches). But they all have one thing in common: They are broken down into glucose, the body's primary fuel. As carbohydrates are digested, glucose is released into the bloodstream. This signals specialized cells in the pancreas to secrete insulin, which is also released into the blood.

Insulin is a nutritional storage hormone. Without it, glucose circulating in the bloodstream cannot enter the cells and be burned for energy. Like a key, insulin opens the cell doors and allows glucose in. As soon as glucose is cleared from the blood, insulin levels fall. It's an ingenious process that, under normal circumstances, proceeds like clockwork every time you eat. But as we've discussed, the massive quantities of carbohydrates we've been consuming over the past 25 years are not normal circumstances.

The amount of insulin released by the pancreas is directly related to the amount of glucose in the blood. If a lot of glucose enters the bloodstream at once, a correspondingly large amount of insulin is required to clear it out. Our systems are not designed to handle great influxes of glucose. When you base your diet on dense, rapidly absorbed carbohydrates that quickly flood the bloodstream with glucose, you are overtaxing your blood sugar regulating system—and this can have disastrous consequences for weight and other health issues.

Carbohydrates have traditionally been lumped into two main categories: simple and complex. Simple carbohydrates like white sugar are so named because they contain only one or two simple sugars, while grains, tubers, and vegetables, made up of longer chains of sugars, are considered complex. The old school of thought figured that simple carbs, such as sugars, should only be eaten in limited quantities, while complex carbs were carte blanche because they would have less of an impact on blood glucose levels. That's how, back in the low-fat heyday, we justified our recommendations for basing meals around baked potatoes, rice, and whole wheat bread.

Once again, we were wrong. When someone finally got around to testing this theory in the early 1980s, the old paradigm was shattered and the new concept of the glycemic index was born. What we learned is that most vegetables, legumes, and fruits do indeed promote a slow and sustained release of blood sugar. These foods have a low glycemic index. Starchy carbohydrates such as potatoes, rice, and bread, on the other hand, have a high glycemic index, meaning they rapidly drive blood sugar up—even more than simple carbohydrates like white sugar. But it gets even more complicated. Any given food may have different effects depending on its form. Whole fruit, for example, stimulates a more gradual and sustained response than fruit juice and thus has a lower glycemic index. Whole oats have quite a different effect on blood sugar than highly processed instant oatmeal. And all those low-fat, refined grain products that have become a major part of our diet send blood sugar and insulin levels soaring.

WHY EXCESS CARBS MAKE YOU F...

Where does this all fit into weight loss? First, those extra dai...
for men and 335 for women—that have sneaked into the ty...
diet in the form of carbohydrates over the past 20 years are not...
at. If you do nothing to burn off these additional calories, weight gain is inevitable.

But I think the more important question is *why* we're eating all those excess calories. A major problem with consuming high-glycemic carbohydrates is that they make you hungry. It's true—eating can make you hungry. When you grab, say, a bagel and orange juice for breakfast, it is quickly digested and absorbed, and you get an enormous rush of blood glucose. This is followed by a correspondingly large release of insulin, which is required to clear all that glucose from the blood. But this sizeable infusion of insulin often works too well, and within a couple of hours your blood sugar level falls even lower than it was before you ate. Your brain, your body's single largest user of glucose, picks up on even minute decreases in its favored fuel. After all, maintaining a constant supply of glucose is a well-honed survival mechanism. So your brain does two things to restore normal blood sugar levels. It triggers the release of hormones such as epinephrine (best known as a stress hormone) to mobilize stored glucose, and it sends out powerful signals to get more glucose into the system.

These hunger messages are not telling you to eat eggs or salad. The brain is specifically crying out for a quick fix of glucose, which is found in the same high-glycemic carbohydrates that caused the problem in the first place. So you hit the break room at work or raid the pantry for a muffin, candy bar, or even whole wheat crackers, and you start the process over again. If you've had trouble in the past staying on a low-fat diet, now you know why. You think you're doing the right thing by eating more low-fat, high-carbohydrate foods, but you just can't resist overeating. It's not your fault. You don't rationally decide that you're going to have that handful of pretzels or that doughnut. Low blood sugar makes you do it.

There's another dark side of elevated insulin. Although many people know that this hormone moves glucose into the cells, few realize that it also regulates fat metabolism and storage. Without insulin, your body cannot ore fat. One of the hallmarks of patients with untreated type 1 diabetes, which is caused by an inability of the pancreas to produce adequate insulin, is weight loss. There is simply not enough insulin to usher nutrients into the cells. People with type 1 diabetes are often ravenously hungry and may eat all the time, but they continue to lose weight.

Too much insulin, on the other hand, *causes* weight gain. When insulin is released into the blood, where it remains for several hours after eating carbohydrates, you burn glucose for energy and store fat. After your energy needs are met, extra glucose is converted into glycogen and deposited in the liver and muscles for future use. When these storehouses are full, whatever additional glucose is floating around in the blood is converted into fat and escorted by insulin into your fat cells.

The weighty effects of too much insulin can clearly be seen in insulin-dependent diabetics. An excess of insulin in the bloodstream encourages weight gain by both increasing appetite (again, overshooting the mark and causing low blood sugar and carbohydrate cravings) and promoting fat storage. At the same time, excess body fat impairs insulin's ability to lower blood sugar, worsening the diabetic condition and setting up a vicious cycle that cascades into all sorts of problems.

I remember a patient who came to the clinic a few years ago with a 10-year history of type 2 diabetes. When he was first diagnosed he was started on an oral drug that stimulates insulin production. It worked for a while, but over the next few months, both his blood sugar and his weight increased. His doctor upped his medication dose, he gained more weight, and his blood sugars climbed higher. After a while, the drug was no longer able to control his diabetes, so he was started on a low dose of insulin. Every few months he returned to his doctor, who kept increasing his dose of insulin to keep his blood sugar under control. And every visit he continued to gain weight. This went on for 10 years, and during that time he gained 100 pounds!

When I first saw this patient, he was taking a hefty 100 units of insulin, yet he was still having problems with blood sugar control. After reviewing his history, completing a physical exam, and evaluating his blood chemistry, I stopped his insulin completely because I knew it was contributing to his multiple health problems. In fact, his diabetes, marked obesity, and high blood fats were all "doctor induced." His treatment: Undo what his previous doctors had done. Over the next few years, this patient lost the 100 pounds he had gained, and his blood sugar fell into the normal range, without diabetic medication.

There's one more insulin issue relating to weight gain I want to mention briefly. If you tend to put on pounds around your abdomen, you likely have insulin resistance, and a high carbohydrate diet may be your worst enemy. That's because the muscle, fat, and liver cells of people with this condition, which affects up to 40 percent of the population, are resistant to insulin's signals. When they eat starches and sugars, the pancreas responds by churning out more and more insulin, "knocking" louder and louder on the doors of the cells in an effort to get all that glucose inside. In addition to affecting appetite and fat storage, a chronically high blood level of insulin also increases triglycerides and lowers protective HDL cholesterol. It raises blood pressure and damages the arteries. Metabolic syndrome, as this collection of problems is known, is a stepping stone to heart disease and especially to type 2 diabetes.

By following the Whitaker Wellness Weight Loss Program and changing the types of carbohydrates you consume, you will return to the diet your body is designed to eat. You will eliminate wild blood sugar swings and elevations in insulin. You will say goodbye to near-constant hunger and carbohydrate cravings. You will restore your body's normal fat burning and storage mechanisms and increase your cells' sensitivity to insulin. And, without exception, you will lose weight.

John, who hails from Dallas, Texas, weighed 235 pounds when he first came to the clinic in June 2005. A smoker and drinker for many years, he admittedly had little discipline when it came to diet and exercise. Like you, he knew what he needed to do, but he just never seemed to get around to doing it. This time, something clicked, and John returned home with a firm resolve to go the distance on the Whitaker Wellness Weight Loss Program. When he came back to the clinic three months later and 31 pounds lighter, he reported, "I realized it was up to me to make the change. I went home and put your suggestions into effect, and the weight just started melting off. Now, I eat to live rather than live to eat."

Ryan, who is in his mid-twenties, lost 60 pounds in two and a half years by avoiding fast food and sweets. Jack, who had lost weight in the past, only to gain it back, dropped 30 pounds—and his blood pressure and cholesterol returned to normal. I personally have lost 25 pounds on the Whitaker Wellness Weight Loss Program, and you can too.

IN ADDITION TO INSULIN . . .

Although insulin is the focus of this chapter, it is not the only hormone that affects weight. Leptin, adiponectin, resistin, ghrelin, cholecystokinin, and the recently discovered obestatin have also been shown to influence appetite and fat storage. The pace of research into these and other hormones has picked up dramatically in recent years. Scientists are trying to gain a better understanding of them and their influences on weight, and they are being explored as targets for weight loss drugs. Some day, one of them may indeed turn out to be a magic bullet for weight loss. But for now, the only thing you can do to reduce your fat stores is good old-fashioned diet and exercise.

4

BEYOND CARBOHYDRATES

Although I am convinced that the number one cause of our epidemic of obesity is our unprecedented intake of sugars and starches, there are obviously other things underlying weight gain. We all know those lucky people who never gain a pound, despite eating lots of bread, pasta, and cookies, and know others who seem to be unable to lose weight no matter how hard they try.

Obesity is a complex phenomenon influenced by a tapestry of genetic, physical, social, and behavioral factors. Let's take a look at some of these other factors and what you can do about them.

DO YOUR GENES MAKE YOU FAT?

As in every facet of heath, heredity plays a role in weight. Children of heavy parents tend to be overweight, and it's not uncommon to see entire families in which virtually all the members are either lean or heavy. Scientists have been looking for a "fat gene" for years. And while they've found several candidates that appear to contribute to weight gain, it is highly unlikely that a single gene causes weight gain.

As I hope I made clear in the last chapter, human beings are not equipped to handle large amounts of sugars and starch. Only in recent history have these foods been available for consumption, and our digestive and endocrine systems never developed the ability to properly metabolize large influxes of rapidly absorbed carbohydrates. This doesn't mean our genes are defective. Our bodies work great when we eat vegetables, fruits, protein, and natural fats—the foods our ancestors have eaten for millennia. Most of us can handle limited amounts of starches and sugars, but when our genome clashes with our environment, i.e., an overabundance of high-glycemic carbohydrates, we're in for big trouble.

This is most dramatically illustrated by the Pima Indians living on reservations near Phoenix, Arizona. About 70 percent of the Pima are obese, and more than half of the adults have diabetes. This is because something in their genotype, sometimes referred to as a "thrifty gene," makes their bodies highly efficient at storing fat. Does this mean the Pima Indians are somehow genetically inferior? Heck, no. They are descendants of nomadic hunters who survived for centuries in the harsh terrain of the Southwest. This inherited trait kept them alive through droughts, famines, and other hardships. But when you plop them down in the land of potato chips and 25-ounce sodas, this once-favorable trait works against them.[1]

This genetic predisposition towards storing fat does not destine all Pimas to being overweight and having diabetes. Close relatives of the Arizona Pimas living in Mexico share the same genome but have none of their medical problems. That's because they live in an environment similar to that of centuries past. They engage in strenuous labor and eat a traditional diet. The culprit here is not just genetics but the interaction of genes and environment.

So while your genes don't *make* you fat, several inherited traits make it easier for some people to maintain normal weight than others under the same environmental conditions. One is basic body type. Some people are naturally thin with wiry muscles and relatively few fat cells. These people have slight, narrow frames and little capacity for body fat storage. Fashion models and marathon runners tend to have this body type. At the opposite end of the spectrum are those whose bodies are rounder, denser, and more muscular. They have more fat cells, bigger muscles, and a greater fat storage capacity—picture NFL linemen. Most people fall somewhere in between, but it's easy to see we're not all working with the same body type. The more fat cells you have, the easier it is to gain weight.

Also, where you gain weight is genetically programmed. Fat is stored in billions of adipose (fat) cells located throughout your body, but we don't all store it in the same area. The most visible type of fat is subcutaneous fat, which is located just below the skin. Love handles, cellulite on the thighs, and any fat you can grab and shake are prime examples. The other type is visceral adipose tissue (VAT), which lies beneath the muscles and around the organs. A big belly, even on someone who is not otherwise overweight, is a sign of excessive VAT. Gender is partly responsible for fat distribution: men tend to deposit fat around their midsection, women in the buttocks and thighs. But again, whether or not you actually gain weight in your belly or your butt is a consequence of both genetic and environmental influences.

Accept the fact that weight maintenance is not an even playing field. It's easier for some people than it is for others. On the other hand, don't blame your weight problems on dear old mom and dad. Your genetic makeup may predispose you towards weight gain, but your behavior, your eating habits, and your activity levels are completely under your control.

Take a hard look at yourself and your close family members, acknowledge what you've got to work with, and don't set yourself up for failure with unrealistic expectations. No amount of dieting or exercising can turn everyone into a supermodel or a ripped weightlifter. No matter how hard I try, I will never be skinny. I have broad shoulders and a muscular, stocky build—big-boned, my wife kindly says. I also have a tendency to put on weight around the midsection. My stepdaughter, on the other hand, is a waif, 5 feet 1 inch and 100 pounds soaking wet. She may gain a few pounds in her hips (which, of course, she thinks makes her fat), but this young woman just doesn't have much fat storage capacity. That's genetics. But gaining 20 or 30 excess pounds? That's environment.

THE SKINNY ON FAT AND MEDICAL CONDITIONS

Most patients who come to the Whitaker Wellness Institute don't come primarily for weight loss. They come with a plethora of health problems from heart disease and diabetes to arthritis and menopause. But the majority of them share a common desire: They want to lose weight. I can't tell you how many times over the past 30 years I've been told by patients that something unique about their medical history makes them unable to lose weight.

The reality is, in most cases, their weight has contributed to their health problems, not the other way around. Obesity pokes its fat fingers into just about every system in the body. As we discussed in Chapter 1, being over-weight increases your risk of heart disease, high cholesterol, hypertension, diabetes, insulin resistance, arthritis, and many other serious conditions. You have no idea how often these diseases improve—and in many cases dis-appear—once weight is brought under control.

That said, let's look at some of the medical conditions that may exacer-bate weight gain. The most significant, in addition to insulin resistance and diabetes, which we've already covered, is hypothyroidism, or low thyroid. The thyroid, a butterfly-shaped gland that wraps around the windpipe, secretes hormones that regulate the body's metabolic rate. When the thyroid is overactive and produces too many hormones, things speed up. Body tem-perature, heart rate, and bowel activity increase. You feel wired and irritable and may have trouble sleeping. More energy is burned, so fat and protein stores are mobilized and weight is lost. Conversely, when thyroid hormone output is low, everything slows down. Body temperature drops, and you feel cold, especially in the extremities. The gastrointestinal system becomes slug-gish, and you may be overcome with fatigue. Because the cells use less energy, weight is gained, even though appetite is often poor.

Undiagnosed hypothyroidism is unbelievably common. According to a recent study, it affects 10 percent of Americans, most of them women, yet the majority doesn't know they have it. If you suspect you have low thyroid, ask your doctor for a thyroid stimulating hormone (TSH) test. TSH is a pituitary hormone that acts like an on/off switch, regulating the secretion of thyroid hormones. When levels of TSH are abnormally high, it means that the thyroid is underactive and is not producing adequate amounts of hormones.

If you are diagnosed with hypothyroidism, you'll probably be treated with Synthroid (levothyroxine), a synthetic version of the T_4 thyroid hor-mone. That, in my opinion, is a mistake. The thyroid gland produces a num-ber of hormones, and it only makes sense to supplement with the whole gamut. I've seen many patients over the years have dramatic improvements in symptoms, including weight, after starting on natural thyroid replace-ment therapy.

One of them was Joyce. When she turned 52, she felt her life was falling apart. Gone was the energetic, upbeat, avid exerciser who had always maintained her ideal weight of 145. In its place was a tired, depressed woman who couldn't keep her weight down. She was diagnosed with hypothyroidism and started on Synthroid. After two years on this drug, she was more fatigued, depressed, and heavier than ever. Once she switched to Armour natural thyroid, however, things turned around.

"It was the difference between night and day," she said. "The very first day, I noticed the difference in how I was feeling. I just got better and better every day. I started to feel like a normal person, like the person I used to be. My weight had kept creeping up slowly, and this bothered me terribly, as I have always been weight-conscious and exercised. I started to lose weight and began a diet with 20 minutes of walking a day. I am happy to report I've lost 21 pounds and know that I will lose more."

You can get a pretty good idea of your thyroid function by the old tried-and-true method of underarm basal (resting) temperature testing. All you need is a thermometer. A basal thermometer with more marked gradations, which is available at any drugstore, is preferable, but a regular thermometer will do.

Shake the thermometer down at night before you go to sleep and keep it at your bedside. First thing in the morning, while you're still in bed and before you move around, put it under your armpit for exactly 10 minutes. Record your temperature. Repeat this process for four days, then average the four readings. (Women who are menstruating should note that only temperatures taken on the first through fourth day of their cycle are accurate.) Normal readings are between 97.8 and 98.2. Temperatures consistently under 97.8 degrees suggest inadequate thyroid production. If yours is low, ask your doctor to confirm hypothyroidism with a TSH test. Even if your TSH is in the low-normal range, I recommend that you request a therapeutic trial of natural thyroid hormone replacement. It could make all the difference in the world.

Deficiencies in other hormones may also affect weight. Many women report weight gain at menopause, but we're not sure if it's caused by a decrease in hormones or if it's simply related to aging. There is a definite tendency for both men and women to put on weight as they get older. Metabolism slows down, lean body mass declines, and fat distribution increases in the abdomen and buttocks. Testosterone, which declines in men just as estrogen and progesterone decline in women, may not directly affect weight either, but it certainly affects muscle. Reduced testosterone leads to muscle wasting and increased accumulation of belly fat. I'm a big fan of *natural* hormone replacement therapy, which, unlike the most popular brands of prescription hormones, are identical to those produced by the human body. (They are available by prescription through compounding pharmacies.) I prescribe natural estrogen, progesterone, and testosterone for many of my older patients not for weight loss per se but to improve many of the signs and symptoms of aging.

Another hormone that declines with age in both men and women and may contribute to weight gain is dehydroepiandrosterone (DHEA). Produced by the adrenal glands, DHEA is a precursor to estrogen, testosterone, and other hormones. Levels in the blood peak around age 20, then fall as we age. Hundreds of studies link declines in DHEA levels with a number of age-related health problems, including abdominal obesity and insulin resistance, and recent research suggests that supplemental DHEA retards the accumulation of abdominal fat. (See Chapter 9 for details.)

You may have heard that cortisol, a hormone released in response to stress, causes obesity. While chronically elevated cortisol levels may have some effect on fat stores, especially in the abdominal area, contrary to advertised claims it's not a primary cause of obesity. There is a disease called Cushing's syndrome caused by exceptionally high levels of cortisol that leads to fat deposits in the upper body and around the neck and back. However, it's quite rare and an infrequent cause of weight gain.

Patients also express concern that their drugs make them fat, and it's true that some drugs do. Insulin, as I told you in the last chapter, most certainly encourages weight gain, and when patients with type 2 diabetes start using insulin, weight gain is almost guaranteed. Oral diabetic drugs that stimulate insulin production, including Glucotrol, DiaBeta, and other sulfonylureas, often cause patients to put on pounds as well. Avandia and Actos, which belong to a class of diabetic drugs called thiazolidinediones, are also problematic because they increase the number of fat cells and stimulate appetite by affecting leptin levels. (This is only one of the reasons I take diabetic patients off all oral drugs.)

Prednisone, a corticosteroid used to reduce inflammation, is notorious for causing rapid weight gain. Half of the patients taking this drug daily put on as much as 28 pounds in just one year. Beta blockers, prescribed for patients with heart disease or hypertension, may lower basal metabolic rate and cause fatigue, resulting in decreased activity and increased weight. Many women believe that oral contraceptives and hormone replacement therapy make them heavier. However, this is not supported by research.

Finally, a wide range of psychotropic drugs are linked with weight gain. These include drugs to treat schizophrenia, bipolar disorder, seizures, anxiety, and depression. The wildly popular selective serotonin reuptake inhibitors (SSRIs), such as Prozac, Paxil, and Zoloft, may cause weight loss at first, but over the long term, they frequently have the opposite effect. This is not surprising because these drugs affect serotonin, a neurotransmitter that affects not only mood but also appetite.

If you are taking any of the drugs listed above, talk to your doctor about non-drug solutions. At the Whitaker Wellness Institute, we routinely take patients off drugs and replace them with safe, effective, natural therapies. This, in combination with the Whitaker Wellness Weight Loss Program diet and exercise regimen, has enabled thousands of patients not only to lose significant amounts of weight but to get well.

SLEEP AND OBESITY

Could insomnia be contributing to your weight problem? According to a survey of more than 9,000 Americans, people who get four hours of sleep or less a night are 73 percent more likely to become obese than those who sleep seven to nine hours per night. According to a study by Columbia University and the Obesity Research Center, even getting six hours—which is pretty normal by today's standards—increases risk of obesity by 27 percent.[2]

When animals and humans are deprived of REM sleep (the most restful and rejuvenating stage), they tend to overeat. Scientists believe this is due to imbalances in two hormones that influence eating behavior. Sleep deprivation causes a decrease in levels of leptin, which dampens appetite, and an increase in levels of ghrelin, an appetite stimulant. Some researchers have theorized that this is a carryover from our distant past when the short nights of summer stimulated an increase in appetite to store fat for the long winter ahead.

Another link between sleep and weight is sleep apnea, the periodic cessation of breathing caused by partial or complete blockage of the airway during sleep. People with sleep apnea fail to get adequate REM sleep, and this wreaks havoc on their health. Sleep apnea adversely affects glucose and insulin metabolism, impairs insulin sensitivity, and increases risk of diabetes five-fold. It also triples risk of hypertension and is an independent risk factor for heart disease, stroke, atrial fibrillation, and heart failure. Erectile problems, cancer, immune dysfunction, memory loss, concentration difficulties . . . the list of problems associated with sleep apnea goes on and on.

Obesity is very closely associated with sleep apnea, and weight loss is an effective treatment for this condition. On the other hand, heavy people who have been treated for sleep apnea often find it easier to control appetite and lose weight. If you snore heavily and you're overweight—having a 17-inch neck (16 inches in women) is a clear warning sign—you have sleep apnea, and you need to do something about it.

"MY METABOLISM IS TOO SLOW"

Have you ever felt like your metabolism is just too slow, that you don't burn calories like other people do? You could be right. Your weight is obviously dependent on how many calories you burn, and some people do have lower metabolic rates than others. About 70 percent of the energy your body uses goes towards maintaining your basic physiological demands: the pumping of the blood, breathing, and maintaining body temperature. Your basal metabolic rate (BMR, also called resting metabolic rate) is the minimum number of calories you need to stay alive while at rest.

Computing your BMR involves a rather complicated mathematical formula based on weight, height, age, and gender that I won't go into here. But to give you an idea, the BMR of a 30-year-old, 5-foot-10-inch man who weighs 180 pounds is 1,870 calories. A 5-foot-5-inch, 140-pound, 45-year-old woman's BMR is 1,334 calories.

Several things affect your basal metabolic rate. One is how much muscle tissue you have. Muscles are loaded with mitochondria, your cells' energy-producing factories where sugars and fats are burned, so the more lean muscle mass, the higher the BMR. Men's BMRs are higher than women's because they naturally have more muscle and less body fat. Younger people's BMRs are also higher for the same reason. Tall people have higher BMRs than short people, simply because they have more body surface area to maintain.

On top of these usual variables, some people are just born with faster metabolism. They have a higher BMR, burn more calories even when they're sleeping, and tend to be thin. Others have BMRs lower than expected, which is associated with a tendency to gain weight. (Those darn genes again.)

You can increase your BMR by adding more muscle mass, and the way to do this is engaging in muscle-building activity. That's why weight training exercise is an important part of the Whitaker Wellness Weight Loss Program. You can lose weight on this diet without exercising, but if you want to keep the pounds off with less effort in the long run, you need to increase your basal metabolic rate. As you add more muscle, you'll burn more calories even when you're just sitting around.

I also recommend that you avoid very low-calorie dieting. When you severely restrict your food intake, your body goes into starvation mode. In an effort to conserve fat stores, it begins breaking down lean muscle tissue for some of its energy needs. This loss of muscle mass can reduce BMR by as much as 20 percent. Individuals who frequently go on low-calorie crash diets without incorporating exercise into their weight loss program end up with very poor body composition (low ratio of muscle to fat) and a depressed BMR.

BURN, BABY, BURN

The calories you burn beyond those required to keep you alive is where the rubber really meets the road, because this is an area over which you have complete control. Physical activity accounts for somewhere between 20 and 40 percent of calories burned daily. The range is so great because our activity levels are so varied. If you sit at a desk all day you obviously use less energy than if you climb stairs and carry heavy loads at a construction site.

You may be surprised by how many calories you burn through your usual daily activities. An hour of housecleaning eats up 200 to 300 calories, and vigorous gardening uses 300 to 400. Even little things such as crossing and uncrossing your legs, standing up, stretching, walking across a room, and maintaining good posture require energy. These small movements, which you may dismiss as trivial in terms of activity, are known as non-exercise activity thermogenesis, or NEAT. Thermogenesis is defined as the generation of heat in the body. It's an index of how much energy or calories the body is using. And NEAT, which does not include formal exercise and intentional activity, can be a significant form of caloric expenditure and weight control.

Some individuals burn hundreds of calories a day through NEAT. These are the people you likely think of as fidgety. I work with one of them. Although she does most of her work at a desk and her job would be considered sedentary, she moves around all the time. When she talks on the phone, she's always standing up, stretching her legs, or fiddling with something. She jumps up a couple of times an hour to get a drink of water or refill her coffee cup, and she doesn't walk down the hall, she strides. In meetings she jiggles her foot and squirms around in her chair. And despite the fact that this girl can eat, she is thin as a rail. I'm not suggesting we should all become fidgeters, but these seemingly inconsequential activities do make a difference, and we can all make an effort to move around more during the course of the day.

Of course, the best way to burn more calories and encourage fat loss is to engage in physical exercise. Most people's notion of exercise is aerobic exercise, such as fast walking, jogging, swimming, cycling, and other fast-paced activities. The benefits of aerobic exercise are undeniable, and I strongly endorse it. Less well recognized are the benefits of weight training. We lose more than six pounds of lean muscle mass per decade of life after our twenties, a loss that accelerates after age 45. While some of this decline is simply a matter of age, the more important reason is because we don't use our muscles. One and only one thing restores muscle mass: weight training and other types of resistance exercise.[3]

If you've exercised in the past and felt it made no difference in your weight, prepare to be very pleasantly surprised on the Whitaker Wellness Weight Loss Program. My exercise regimen, which is laid out for you in a step-by-step plan in Chapter 10, is not an entity in and of itself. It is designed to work in conjunction with the diet. As I explained in the previous chapter, when you eat carbohydrates, glucose is released into your bloodstream. If you exercise after eating carbohydrates, you'll burn these carbs for fuel. However, when you restrict your carb intake, fat is mobilized out of your fat cells and used for energy. In other words, on the Whitaker Wellness Weight Loss Program diet, you'll turn on your body's natural fat-burning mechanisms, and if you add exercise, you'll rev them up into high gear.

WHAT YOU EAT AFFECTS HOW MUCH YOU EAT

I want to close this chapter by reiterating my opening message. The primary cause of our weight problem is eating the wrong foods. No doubt about it, we eat too much—an average of 250 calories a day more than we ate 25 years ago. In 1970, the average bagel was three inches in diameter and had 140 calories. Now it's six inches and 350 calories. A soda used to contain 85 calories in a 6.5-ounce bottle. Today's 20-ouncers total 250 calories. And you need only look as far as the nearest restaurant to confirm that portions are bigger than they used to be. A typical plate of spaghetti and meatballs used to have 500 calories; now they've more than doubled at 1,250.

You can blame this on food manufacturers or restaurants for serving up too much food if you want, but they wouldn't be dishing it out if we weren't lapping it up. I don't buy the argument that the American public has become a bunch of lazy, gluttonous pigs in the past 25 years. We're eating more because we're hungry, and we're hungry because the types of food we consume literally compel us to overeat. Government statistics clearly illustrate that most of our 250 extra daily calories are in the form of carbohydrates. When half of your caloric intake comes from starch and sugar, appetite increases and fat burning makes way for fat storage, virtually setting you up for weight gain.

However, if you cut sugars and starches out of your diet, your appetite will easily be tamed, and weight loss will become effortless.

5

WHY THIS
PROGRAM WORKS

Jonathan is a successful businessman who struggled with his weight for years. It wasn't until the scales crept up to 248 pounds that he realized he needed to get serious about weight loss. So three years ago he did something very simple: He cut out breads, pasta, breaded fried foods, and desserts. That's it. He didn't count calories or follow a set meal plan. He didn't start jogging or lifting weights. He just made a commitment to avoid starches and sugars, and what a difference it has made.

Over the course of about a year, Jonathan lost about one pound a week. That may not sound like much, but after a year, he had lost 45 pounds, and today he weighs in at a lean, mean 190.

As Jonathan will attest, the Whitaker Wellness Weight Loss Program works. And once you make the commitment to give it a go, you'll find it's far, far, easier to adhere to than the diets in your past. That's because it encompasses a wide variety of foods that, in addition to helping you lose weight, are tasty and familiar. You will not be required to scour your health food store shelves for ingredients you've never heard of, nor will you have to endure bland, boring meals. You'll also get plenty to eat—I guarantee you won't get up from the table hungry and snacks aren't just allowed, they're encouraged. Furthermore, it's easy. You don't have to obsess about calories or calculate percentages of this or that. All you need to do is eat the recommended foods and avoid those that stimulate weight gain.

Let's take a look at why this program works.

YOU'LL EAT LESS

For starters, because the foods you'll be eating are highly satiating, you'll eat less. Satiety is defined as "the quality or state of being fed or gratified to or beyond capacity." If you eat foods that fill you up and tide you over, you'll be less likely to overeat. I think you know by now which foods are the worst in terms of satiety: starchy and sugary carbohydrates. But what are the best?

Susanna Holt, Ph.D., of the University of Sydney in Australia, conducted a study to quantify the "satiety index" of various foods. She fed 240 calories of 38 different foods to a group of study subjects, then over the next two hours rated their feelings of hunger and observed what they ate from a buffet. Overall, the foods with the highest satiety index were protein-rich foods, with high-fiber carbohydrate foods coming in second. Fatty foods were the least satisfying, most likely because fat tends to be stored rather than immediately used, so it doesn't trigger the satiety signals that tell you to stop eating.[1]

Many other studies point to protein as the star of satiety. Researchers at the University of Washington in Seattle found that when people got 30 percent of their calories from protein and 20 percent from fat, they ate fewer calories than when they were on a 15 percent protein diet—even though they had no restrictions on their food intake. On the higher protein diet, they ate an average of 441 fewer calories per day than when they were consuming less protein, and over 12 weeks, lost an average of 11 pounds.[2]

YOU'LL STORE FEWER CALORIES

Did you know that the mere act of eating burns calories? That's right. Between 5 and 15 percent of your daily energy expenditure is used up digesting, absorbing, and storing food, a type of caloric use referred to as postprandial or diet-induced thermogenesis (DIT). But not all foods burn up the same amount of energy.

When you eat fat, your DIT only goes up 0 to 3 percent. During digestion, dietary fats are broken down by bile acids into tiny particles of fat.

These particles are absorbed by the lymphatic system, released into the bloodstream, and carried to fat cells for storage. It's not as "labor intensive" a process as is required for carbohydrate or protein assimilation, and it doesn't require much energy.

Carbohydrate digestion, absorption, and storage necessitate more work by the body. These nutrients are broken down in the digestive tract into glucose and absorbed into the bloodstream. This stimulates the pancreas to produce insulin, which moves glucose into the cells. If excess glucose is floating around, it must either be converted into glycogen and stored in the liver and muscles, or converted into fat and stored in the adipose cells. More steps, more work, more calories burned. The DIT of carbohydrate is 5 to 10 percent.

The clear winner in postprandial thermogenesis (burning up calories in the digestion process) is protein. Protein is broken down by the digestive system into amino acids, which are released into the bloodstream. The body uses amino acids to make new proteins for tissue building and to create enzymes, hemoglobin, hormones, and other functional proteins. Unlike fats and carbohydrates, proteins are not stored. Some are converted into metabolic fuels and used as energy, but most excess proteins are broken down into uric acid and urea and excreted in the urine. This takes a lot of energy and burns 20 to 30 percent of calories ingested. According to a 2004 Dutch review of 15 studies, postprandial thermogenesis of a high-protein/low-fat diet is twice as high as a high-carbohydrate/low-fat diet.[3]

As an aside (we'll return to this later) alcohol also has a hefty DIT: 10 to 30 percent, which is much higher than fat and carbohydrates and almost as high as protein. That's one reason why the Whitaker Wellness Weight Loss Program does not forbid alcohol. Of course, alcohol must be used in moderation, but a drink a day is associated with increased insulin sensitivity and lower weight.

YOU'LL BURN FAT

Burning fat is obviously important for weight loss, and you can turn on your body's fat-burning mechanisms by eating the right types of food. The preferred high-octane fuel of the body is carbohydrate in the form of glucose.

Between meals, when there's no fresh supply of glucose in your blood, energy is derived from glycogen, which is stored in the liver and muscles. Once these limited stores are used up—and they're exhausted quite rapidly—the body starts burning fat.

When you get out of bed in the morning, your body is burning fat, because the eight to 12 hours between dinner and breakfast are ample time to have depleted your glucose stores. Then you eat Shredded Wheat and an English muffin with jam for breakfast, which sends your blood glucose and insulin levels soaring. This shuts down the mobilization and burning of fat, and your body shifts over to burning glucose and storing fat. If you eat cookies and crackers for snacks and pasta and rice at mealtime, you'll go through the whole day burning glucose, and the only time you'll ever use fat for energy is when you're sleeping.

However, if you do not introduce significant amounts of glucose into your system by avoiding high-glycemic carbohydrates for breakfast, you will continue to burn fat through the morning. If you snack on nuts or cottage cheese and eat ample amounts of protein and green vegetables at meals, you'll remain in the fat-burning mode all day long. Your body will run fine on this alternative energy source. Burning fat is normal—it's what kept us alive in times of famine and what allows people to fast for extended periods.

If you've heard that it's dangerous, that's because there's a tremendous amount of confusion about a byproduct of fat-burning called ketosis, or the presence of ketones in the blood. When fats are mobilized into the bloodstream, carbon compounds called ketones, or ketone bodies, are synthesized in the liver. Ketosis is perfectly safe. In fact, ketones are an exceptionally efficient fuel, second only to glucose. Concerns arise when ketosis gets mixed up with ketoacidosis, a decidedly dangerous condition that can occur in uncontrolled diabetes. Characterized by very high concentrations of ketones in the blood that upset the body's acid-base balance, ketoacidosis can be fatal if untreated. Run-of-the-mill ketosis involves much lower levels of ketones, and its only downside is that, because ketones that aren't used for energy are expelled through the lungs and urine, they can make your breath smell funny.

In summary, the Whitaker Wellness Weight Loss diet will enable you to eat less and burn fat—a winning combo for weight loss.

HIGH-QUALITY PROTEIN

Since protein satiates and burns brightly, it is front and center on the Whitaker Wellness Weight Loss Program. But that doesn't mean this is a high-protein diet. True, I recommend that all your meals and snacks include protein, but in moderate-sized portions. Your average meal will contain 20 to 25 grams of protein—a little less if your frame is small or a little more if you're big. For breakfast, this might be a hearty three-egg omelet (a combination of a whole egg and several egg whites). For lunch and dinner, four ounces of fish, chicken, or lean beef (a serving slightly larger than a deck of cards or the palm of your hand) will hit this protein target. And for snacks, you'll get your protein from a handful of nuts, a hardboiled egg, or a little cottage cheese or peanut or almond butter.

The thing to remember when you're selecting your protein is that no nutrient is an island. Food in its natural state doesn't come in neatly labeled packages of 100 percent protein, fat, or carbohydrate. As the chart below illustrates, most foods are mixtures of these macronutrients, with varying amounts of vitamins, minerals, and other micronutrients thrown in. To reap the benefits of this diet, you must pay attention to the whole package.

It's surprisingly easy. Chicken and turkey with the skin removed, fish, shellfish, and seafood, and lean cuts of beef, lamb, and pork are primarily protein and are excellent choices. They contain no carbohydrate at all and limited amounts of fat. Untrimmed, marbled cuts of meat, however, are loaded with fat. A four-ounce serving of prime rib, for example, has almost twice the fat of a similar-sized serving of trimmed sirloin steak. A chicken thigh contains almost five times more fat and one-third less protein than skinless breast.

Eggs are another good choice, especially egg whites, which are essentially pure protein. The yolk of an egg also contains protein, but it is wrapped up with four grams of fat. There's nothing wrong with eating an egg yolk or two a day; in fact, I recommend it. Even cardiologists now give egg yolks the thumbs-up, recognizing that moderate amounts do not increase risk of heart disease. Yolks are an excellent source of brain-nurturing choline, vision-enhancing lutein, and other important nutrients. Omega-3-enriched

Macronutrient Content of Selected Foods

Food	Portion	Calories	grams Carbohydrate	grams Protein	grams Fat	grams Fiber
All-Bran cereal	¾ cup	119	34	5	1	15
Almonds	¼ cup	209	7	7	19	4
Bagel	1 whole	245	48	9	1	2
Beef, prime rib	4 ounces	338	0	19	28	0
Beef, sirloin, trimmed	4 ounces	229	0	21	16	0
Broccoli, cooked	¾ cup	33	6	3	0	3
Bread, whole wheat	1 slice	69	13	3	1	2
Cabbage, raw	1 cup	22	5	1	0	2
Cashews	¼ cup	187	9	5	16	2
Celery, raw	3 stalks	19	4	1	0	2
Chicken breast, without skin	4 ounces	142	0	27	3	0
Chicken thighs,	4 ounces	189	0	15	14	0
Cheddar cheese,	1 ounce	114	0	7	9	0
Cheddar cheese, reduced fat	1 ounce	49	1	7	2	0
Coconut, unsweetened	2 Tbsp.	159	7	2	15	4
Cottage cheese, fat free	¾ cup	105	5	22	0	0
Cucumber	1 cup	13	3	1	0	1
Egg	1	66	1	5	4	0
Egg whites	2	33	1	7	0	0
Flaxseed	3 tablespoons	165	9	6	13	8
Ground turkey	4 ounces	169	0	20	0	0
Kidney beans, cooked	½ cup	112	20	8	0	6
Lettuce, romaine	1 cup	8	1	1	0	1
Milk, fat-free	1 cup	86	12	8	0	0
Milk, whole	1 cup	150	11	8	8	0
Oatmeal, cooked	¾ cup	104	18	4	2	3
Orange	1 whole	62	15	1	0	3
Orange juice	1 cup	112	26	2	0	0
Peanuts	¼ cup	214	8	9	18	3
Peas, cooked	¾ cup	88	15	6	0	6
Pork tenderloin	4 ounces	136	0	24	4	0
Salmon fillet	4 ounces	132	0	23	4	0
Salsa	¼ cup	18	4	1	0	0
Soybeans, cooked	½ cup	149	9	14	8	5

Food	Portion	Calories	grams Carbohydrate	grams Protein	grams Fat	grams Fiber
Spaghetti, cooked	¾ cup	148	30	5	1	2
Stevia	2 drops	0	0	0	0	0
Tofu	4 ounces	86	2	9	5	1
Tomato	1 med.	26	6	1	0	1
Snickers	1 bar	140	18	2	7	0
Turkey, skinless white meat	4 ounces	122	0	27	1	0
Xylitol	1 tsp	10	4	0	0	0

eggs are even better because they also contain a hefty serving of the omega-3 fatty acids we'll discuss below. But as a source of lean protein, egg whites, either from whole eggs or the egg-white products you'll find in your grocery store, are far superior.

Then there is dairy. Not only are certain dairy products a great way to get protein, but they also contain significant amounts of calcium, which has been shown to facilitate weight loss. (More on this in Chapter 8.) A cup of milk has a reasonable amount of protein, about eight grams, but it also has an equivalent amount of fat and 11 grams of carbohydrate; skim milk loses the fat but gains one gram of carbohydrate. I don't object to a little milk in your coffee, but I do not recommend it as a beverage. The most protein-dense dairy product is nonfat cottage cheese. One cup gives you more protein than an average serving of fish or poultry with no fat and minimal carbohydrates. Cheese is also high in protein, but since it is also high in fat, I recommend reduced-fat varieties. I strongly suggest purchasing organic dairy foods whenever possible.

Nuts and seeds are powerhouses of nutrition and contain some amounts of protein and carbohydrate, along with liberal amounts of fat. Eating nuts is associated with many health benefits, including decreased risk of diabetes and heart disease. A small handful of almonds, walnuts, peanuts, or sunflower seeds makes a nice, balanced snack, but you do need to monitor portions because nuts and seeds are extremely calorie-dense.[4]

Grains and foods made from refined grains such as bread and pasta have reasonable amounts of protein and little fat, but they are loaded—and I do mean loaded—with carbohydrates. Three-quarters cup of cooked oatmeal, for example has four grams of protein, two grams of fat, and 18 grams of carbohydrate (three of them fiber). A slice of 100 percent whole wheat bread clocks in at three grams of protein and 13 grams of carbohydrate (two grams of fiber). And three-fourths cup of cooked pasta may have five grams of protein, but it also has 30 grams of carbs. These items are obviously not welcomed on the Whitaker Wellness Weight Loss Program.

Likewise, beans and legumes contain decent amounts of protein, but like grain foods, they have two or three times more carbohydrate than protein. This is offset to some degree by their high fiber content, but when you're looking to lower your carbohydrate intake, you need to go easy on beans. One exception is soy. Half a cup of cooked dried soybeans weighs in at 14 grams of protein and nine grams of carbohydrate, with five grams of fiber. Prepared foods made from soy such as burgers and hot dogs are very high in protein and low in fat and carbohydrate.

If you are vegetarian, it is still possible to follow the Whitaker Wellness Weight Loss Program, especially if you eat dairy and eggs. It's more challenging for vegans who strictly avoid foods from all animal sources, but it can be done by including plenty of high-protein soy-based foods and supplementing with protein powder.

WHERE DOES FAT FIT IN?

Fat, the villain that terrorized Americans for 20 years and drove us into the comforting arms of fat-free cookies and rice cakes, turns out to be a pussycat. There is nothing at all intrinsically dangerous about dietary fat. In fact, if you don't get enough fat in your diet, your health will suffer. Back in my high-carbohydrate days, I would occasionally see patients with very dry skin and mental "fog" who, as it turned out, had taken the low-fat diet to an extreme. Once they started getting adequate amounts of fat though diet and fish oil supplements, symptoms resolved.

I believe that the late Robert Atkins, M.D., who received more than his share of both acclaim and notoriety, was certainly on the right track in advocating a low-carbohydrate diet for weight loss. Where he missed the boat, in my opinion, was his wanton embrace of fat. Bacon, ribs, hot dogs, pork rinds: The man never met a fat he didn't like. Had he been more judicious in his dietary fat recommendations, his message about the adverse effects of carbohydrates might have been heard by health authorities. He had a lot to offer 25 years ago when the low-fat, high-carb hysteria began, and if we had listened to him, we would all be better off—and we certainly wouldn't be in the middle of an obesity epidemic!

Two types of fat are, as their name suggests, essential for health: omega-3 and omega-6 essential fatty acids (EFAs). These polyunsaturated fats cannot be manufactured by the body and must be obtained through dietary or supplemental sources. The best-studied omega-3s fatty acids are docosahexaenoic acid (DHA), a dominant fat in the brain, and eicosapentaeonic acid (EPA), which has anti-inflammatory effects and broad benefits for the cardiovascular system and overall health. Nature's richest source of omega-3s are fatty fish such as salmon and tuna, which is why I recommend them as a protein source—you get two health benefits for the price of one. The most abundant fat in vegetables, seeds, and nuts is omega-6, so you'll get plenty of this essential fat on the Whitaker Wellness Weight Loss Program as well.

Another type of fat that I encourage you to include in your diet is monounsaturated fat, the primary fat in olive and canola oil. Olive oil, which has been part of the Mediterranean diet for thousands of years, is particularly healthful and has been shown to protect against heart disease by keeping the arteries flexible and guarding against free radical damage. It should be your oil of choice for sautéing, baking, and grilling. I do not recommend polyunsaturated oils for cooking because they break down when exposed to heat, which unleashes oxidative damage, free radical production, and other harmful byproducts. If you want to use unrefined almond, sunflower, sesame, or another polyunsaturated oil in a salad dressing, fine. Just make sure you purchase quality brands from your health food store, and avoid the processed vegetable oils sold in supermarkets.

Saturated fats are found in meat, dairy products, and tropical oils such as palm and coconut. I urge you to go easy on saturated fat from animal sources. Although they're not as bad as health authorities make them out to be, these fats can raise LDL cholesterol. However, the amount of saturated fat you'll get from eating an egg or two a day, a little cheese, and lean poultry, beef, lamb, and pork is perfectly acceptable.

Interestingly, tropical oils such as coconut and palm contain a different kind of saturated fat: medium-chain fatty acids. These fats are easily digested and, rather than being stored as fat, they are burned as energy, which explains why they are used by patients who have trouble digesting fat and by athletes to enhance fat loss and muscle gain. I particularly like coconut oil, because one of its dominant fatty acids, lauric acid, has a host of health benefits. It has antiviral and antibacterial activity, protects the liver, enhances the immune system, and it doesn't raise cholesterol levels. Because coconut oil is very stable when heated, it also makes an excellent cooking oil, although I must warn you that it makes your food smell like an Almond Joy.

The black sheep of the fat family are trans fats. These harmful fats are created during the hydrogenation process, when liquid polyunsaturated oils are chemically altered to make them solid and stable. These unnatural fats raise LDL cholesterol, lower protective HDL cholesterol, and have been linked to increased risk of heart disease, cancer, diabetes, infertility, and obesity. Harvard researchers estimate that trans fats are responsible for tens of thousands of preventable deaths every year.[5] Read labels carefully (food manufacturers are now required to list trans fat content on labels), and steer clear of foods that have been fried in vegetable oils. The top source of trans fats is French fries and other fried foods, which you aren't going to be eating on the Whitaker Wellness Weight Loss Program anyway.

THE RIGHT CARBOHYDRATES

Now let's look at carbohydrates. I want to make it clear from the start that I am not anti-carb. Although this diet is starch and sugar restricted, the bulk of the foods you will be eating at your meals will contain carbohydrates. That's because it's the dominant nutrient in vegetables which—along with fruits, nuts, and seeds—figure prominently in the Whitaker Wellness Weight Loss Program.

One reason I encourage you to eat these foods is because they are so darn good for you. Plant foods contain an abundance of potassium, an essential mineral that helps control blood pressure. Brightly-colored pro-duce is our richest source of vitamin C, beta-carotene, and other antioxi-dants. Leafy greens supply us with magnesium and calcium, and nuts and seeds are loaded with vitamin E and B-complex vitamins. Vegetables and fruits also contain a vast array of phytonutrients found in no other foods, such as vision-protecting lutein in leafy greens, cancer-preventing indoles in broccoli, and heart-healthy polyphenols in berries and grapes.

Vegetables and other plant foods are also excellent sources of fiber, the indigestible parts of plant cell walls that lower blood sugar and cholesterol, improve gastrointestinal health, and aid in weight loss. As I mentioned above, fiber-rich carbohydrates are among the most satiating of all foods, second only to protein. They're bulky, so they fill your stomach up, and they take longer to eat, so you have time to register satiety signals from your brain. Fiber also retards the rate at which food leaves your stomach, caus-ing a slower, more sustained release of blood sugar, and you know what that means for appetite. I've yet to see a patient who got fat overeating broccoli or romaine lettuce. Fiber is so helpful with weight loss that I encourage you to consider adding supplemental fiber to your diet. (We'll talk more about fiber in Chapters 7 and 9.)

While the Whitaker Wellness Weight Loss Program includes lots of vegetables and lesser amounts of fruit and legumes, it does not allow starchy foods such as potatoes, pasta, tortillas, rice, and bread, or concen-trated sources of sugar such as fruit juice and sweets. That's because these are precisely the foods that cause you to feel hungry, overeat, and store fat.

Starchy potatoes and rice and foods made from refined grains are dense, heavy, and loaded with carbohydrates, and the more carbohydrates you eat, the more dramatic the blood sugar and insulin response. Nearly 90 percent of the starchy foods you consume enter the blood as glucose within a cou-ple of hours after you eat, and if you're trying to curb your appetite and encourage fat burning, that's bad news. Carb count adds up quickly with these foods. A slice of whole wheat bread, a cup of cereal, and a cup of non-fat milk give you almost 45 grams of carbohydrate.

Concentrated sugars, which include not only the obvious candy bars and desserts but also fruit juices and excessive amounts of whole fruit, do a similar number. Add a cup of orange juice to that toast and cereal, and you bump your carbohydrate count up to more than 70 grams—enough to you set up for a day-long cycle of hunger, binging, and fat storage.

The foundation of the Whitaker Wellness Weight Loss Program diet is very simple: Avoid these foods altogether. This will dramatically lower your carbohydrate intake and get you on the path to weight loss. I don't want you to cut back on bread, potatoes, desserts, and juice—I want you to eliminate them. I promise it will be much easier to say no altogether than to tease yourself with a handful of potato chips here and half a bagel there.

LIGHTEN YOUR LOAD

As you achieve your weight loss goals, of course, you can liberalize your diet. You may increase your carbohydrate intake by eating more fruits and beans. Add the occasional bowl of fiber-rich oatmeal. Indulge in a sweet treat from time to time (my favorite is a square of dark chocolate). But do not make the mistake of going back to a steady diet of bread and pasta, Cokes, and candy bars. As I explained in Chapter 4, our epidemic of obesity is caused by our unbridled consumption of refined, concentrated starches and sugars. Once you get out of the habit of eating these foods—and what and how much we eat is in large part habit—you'll be well on your way to permanent weight control. Moreover, you'll feel better, you'll have more energy, and you'll be setting yourself up for a lifetime of good health.

The KISS (keep it simple, stupid) method of carbohydrate selection has just one guideline: Avoid starches and sugars. For those of you who want to get more scientific about it, let's return to the concept of the glycemic index (GI). The glycemic index of a food is a measure of how much it triggers a rise in blood sugar. Foods with a low GI provoke smaller, more gradual elevations and provide a nice, steady supply of glucose and energy. Foods with a high GI, however, prompt undesirable rapid blood sugar spikes, followed by equally dramatic plummets.

Since the GI was first developed in 1981 by David Jenkins, M.D., of the

University of Toronto, more than 750 carbohydrate foods have been scientifically tested and assigned a glycemic index. For the most part, the GI of foods is fairly intuitive. As you would predict, highly processed foods made with flour and sugar have a high GI while most vegetables, beans, fruits, and nuts have a low GI. But some unprocessed foods such as rice, potatoes, watermelon, carrots, beets, whole-grain bread, bananas, and pineapple have a high GI, while some refined foods like pasta have a lower GI.

While the GI is very useful, it does have one peculiarity. The GI of a specific food is determined by feeding volunteers a portion of that food containing 50 grams carbohydrate and, over the course of a few hours, measuring their blood sugar levels at regular intervals. The carbohydrate content of different foods varies widely. A heaping cup of spaghetti, a large baked potato, or two doughnuts each contain about 50 grams of carbohydrate. But to get those same 50 grams, you'd have to eat five cups of carrots, four small oranges, or 10 pounds of spinach.

This inspired Walter Willett, M.D., and his colleagues at the Harvard School of Public Health to expand the concept of the GI into something more practical: the glycemic load (GL). Simply put, GL takes into account quality and quantity. It is determined by both the GI of any given food, plus the amount of available, or net, carbohydrates (fiber and sugar alcohols are excluded) in a standard serving.

The GL has a few surprises: Some foods with a high GI actually have minimal effects on blood sugar levels when eaten in normal quantities, while others with a low GI are potentially problematic. For example, carrots and spaghetti have similar GIs. Yet one large carrot contains only five grams of available carbs because much of it is fiber and water. A cup of heavy, dense spaghetti, however, contains about 40 grams of carbohydrate. Therefore, the two have vastly different GLs of 2 and 16, respectively, and markedly different effects on blood sugar.

	GLYCEMIC INDEX	GLYCEMIC LOAD
Low	55 or under	10 or under
Medium	56-69	11-19
High	70 or above	20 or above

Food	Glycemic Index (GI)	Serving Size	Glycemic Load (GI)
Xylitol	8	2 teaspoons	1
Peanuts	14	4 oz	2
Carrots	47	1 large	2
Peas	48	½ cup	3
Watermelon	72	1 cup	4
Rye Pumpernickel Bread	41	1 large slice	5
Apples	38	1 medium	6
Kidney Beans	28	1 cup	7
Popcorn	72	2 cups	7
Flour Tortilla	30	1 medium	8
All-Bran Cereal	38	1 cup	9
Honey	55	1 tablespoon	9
White Bread	70	1 slice	10
Ice Cream	61	1 cup	10
Corn	60	½ cup	11
Oatmeal	58	1 cup	12
Pizza	30	2 slices	13
Low-Fat Yogurt	33	1 cup	16
Spaghetti	42	1 cup	16
Raisins	62	1 small box	20
French Fries	75	⅔ cup	22
Vanilla Cake with Frosting	42	1 small slice	24
Plain Bagel	72	1 small	25
Baked Potato	85	1 medium	28
Potato Chips	54	4 oz	30
Macaroni and Cheese	64	1 serving	30
Snickers Bar	55	1 bar	35

This chart has been modified with permission from mendosa.com, with additional information from nutritiondata.com/glycemic-index.html.

Hundreds of studies have been conducted on the GI and GL, many of them on the effects of low versus high GI/GL diets on patients with diabetes. One Australian study conducted at the University of Sydney, a meta-analysis of 14 clinical trials involving more than 350 diabetic patients, revealed that a low GI diet improved management of blood sugar levels in a manner "similar to that offered by pharmacological agents that also target postprandial hyperglycemia." In other words, it worked as well as some diabetic drugs.[6] A Harvard study found that overweight women who ate a high GL diet were twice as likely to develop coronary heart disease as their thinner counterparts who consumed low GI foods.[7] High GL diets are also linked to increased risk of gallbladder disease and elevations in triglycerides, cholesterol, and C-reactive protein.

Eating low GL carbohydrates will also help you lose weight. By sticking to low GI/GL carbohydrates, it goes without saying that you will cut out the sugary, starchy foods that activate your appetite and cause you to overeat. Lighten your glycemic load and you'll lighten your weight.

THE BIG PICTURE

Before we move on to what you'll be eating on a daily basis as you lose weight, I want to emphasis that this is a "big picture" diet. As a physician, I am compelled to look beyond mere weight loss to the overall nutritional value and health effects of the foods I recommend. You can purchase all kinds of diet foods in your supermarket: artificial sweeteners, diet sodas, fat-free cookies, sugar-free candy, and on and on ad nauseam. But these fake foods have no place in your diet.

The Whitaker Wellness Weight Loss Program is based on whole, natural foods that are exceptionally nutritious and have proven health benefits. That's why, in addition to helping you slim down and look great, it will improve every aspect of your health.

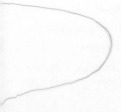

6

THE NUTS AND BOLTS
OF THE DIET

Imagine sitting down to a fillet of salmon grilled to perfection, atop an enormous salad of mixed greens with a tangy dressing. Or a marinated chicken breast with a generous side of asparagus, green beans, or another vegetable of your choice. How about chicken fajitas with plenty of peppers, onions, and guacamole; stir-fried shrimp loaded with vegetables; or a patty melt with cheese and caramelized onions? Chicken Caesar and chef's salad, chili and hearty soups, cheese omelets and vegetable frittatas: These will be your typical meals on the Whitaker Wellness Weight Loss Program.

Easy to prepare, amenable to most everyone's tastes, and adaptable to dining out—you are in for a culinary treat. But what you'll enjoy even more is the ease with which you will lose weight.

Let's get down to the nuts and bolts of the diet.

DON'T SKIP BREAKFAST

You've heard all your life that breakfast is the most important meal of the day, and it makes sense that you need to refuel after an overnight 10- to 12-hour fast. But beyond that, there are lots of good reasons to eat breakfast. Studies spanning several decades show that people who eat breakfast concentrate and learn better. (This is especially true of schoolchildren.) They have more strength and endurance and superior overall nutritional status. Their cholesterol levels are, on average, lower than those of people who skip their morning meal, and their cells are more sensitive to insulin. Furthermore, they are less likely to be obese.

In a study reported in 2005, British researchers tested the effects of eating or forgoing breakfast in a group of healthy, normal-weight women. For two weeks, the women ate bran flakes (very high in fiber and relatively low in available carbohydrates) with 2 percent milk for breakfast, followed by four additional meals or snacks throughout the day. After a two-week break, the women were fed similar meals and snacks, except they skipped breakfast and ate the cereal around noon. The researchers found that during the no-breakfast period, the women's cholesterol levels were higher, their insulin sensitivity was lower, and their appetites were much heartier—they ate an average of 387 extra calories per day![1]

Approximately one-third of Americans routinely skip breakfast, and many do so under the mistaken idea that it helps with weight control. A recent survey showed that almost one in five teenaged girls intentionally avoided breakfast because they believe it will help them slim down. This is nonsense. If you want to lose weight, eat breakfast every day.

Now, what constitutes a healthy breakfast is sorely misunderstood. While it is obvious that doughnuts and Danishes aren't good choices, less apparent is the downside of a whole wheat bagel or a bowl of Corn Flakes. These starchy, high-glycemic carbs, which constitute the typical American breakfast, cause a rapid and dramatic rise in blood sugar levels, followed by a precipitous drop a couple of hours later that can leave you unfocused, irritable, and ravenously hungry. Slow-cooked oatmeal and very high-fiber bran cereals are excellent selections you may enjoy once you've achieved your ideal weight. However, breakfasts on the Whitaker Wellness Weight Loss diet are designed with one thing in mind: to keep you in the fat-burning mode throughout the morning. That's why they're high in protein (20 to 25 grams) and low in carbohydrates (about 10 grams).

If you like eggs, you're going to love this diet. Scrambled, poached, fried, hard-boiled, omelets, frittatas, breakfast quiches: the options are almost endless. You'll hit your protein target by eating three to four large eggs (6 to 7 grams each), six to eight egg whites (3 to 3.5 grams each), or three-fourths to one cup of a liquid egg white product (5 to 6 grams per quarter cup). As we discussed in the previous chapter, I recommend no more than two whole eggs a day, so a combination of whole eggs and egg whites is preferable.

Feel free to add cheese, preferably reduced fat, to your eggs. Each ounce contains seven grams of protein, so use fewer eggs accordingly. You may also swap out three strips of turkey bacon or sausage or an ounce of ham (turkey preferred) for an egg or two egg whites. Lightly sautéed onions, green peppers, mushrooms, and spinach also make eggs more interesting, so feel free to include these and other low-carb vegetables. Not crazy about eggs? Get an equivalent amount of protein from three-fourths cup of nonfat or low-fat cottage cheese or three ounces of turkey, chicken, or reduced-fat cheese. Vegans can substitute equivalent amounts of tofu and other soy products.

Because fruit is so nutritious, I encourage you to have some for breakfast, but be aware that fruits are fairly concentrated sources of carbohydrates, so don't go overboard. We are aiming for around 10 grams of carbohydrate, the amount in a plum, peach, or tangerine; half an apple, orange, nectarine, or grapefruit; or half a cup of blueberries, grapes, or cherries. (See page 127 for a complete list of fruits and acceptable quantities. As for juice, just one cup of orange juice contains 25 grams of carbohydrate. The only acceptable juice on this program is low-sodium V8 Juice (regular V8 has too much salt), and it should be limited to one cup.

If you're just not into breakfast, at least have a meal replacement drink or bar containing 20 to 25 grams of protein and around 10 grams of available carbohydrate. But read labels carefully. Many of the shakes and bars you'll find in your supermarket or health food store contain artificial additives and other unhealthy ingredients—even if they're in the target protein/carbohydrate range.

At first you might miss the toast, bagels, or pancakes you may be used to eating for breakfast, but I promise you won't miss the midmorning blood sugar swings and carbohydrate cravings these starchy carbs cause. In Chapter 14, we've provided lots of menu suggestions and recipes to start your day off with a bang.

LUNCH ON THE GO

Scrounging around in the fridge for leftovers, heating up a microwave meal, making a sandwich, picking up takeout food . . . lunch can be the most problematic meal of the day because it's the one over which you may have the least control. You're at work, so you're unable to go into the kitchen and prepare something healthy. You grab a quick bite at a fast food joint or another restaurant, or you eat the sandwich you hastily threw together before leaving the house. But lunch needn't be a dietary landmine. All it requires is a little planning.

Like breakfast, lunch on the Whitaker Wellness Weight Loss diet will include 20 to 25 grams of lean protein and no more than 10 grams of carbohydrate. You'll get this from a four-ounce serving of lean beef, chicken, turkey, deli meat, tuna or other fish, accompanied by a large salad or side of vegetables.

The easiest lunch is leftovers. I know a lot about leftovers. My wife, Connie, has eight siblings, and between the two of us, we have eight children. When Connie is in the kitchen, she seems to forget that we don't have any kids living at home and cooks enough for a small army. Not that I mind—there's nothing easier than heating up a favorite meal and enjoying it all over again. A big pot of soup provides lunches for days, and when we're tired of it, we freeze it in individual-sized servings for later use.

Salads are another lunchtime favorite. Whether you brown-bag it or order it in a restaurant, a piece of grilled chicken or fish atop a mountain of greens with a tasty dressing makes a satisfying and nutritious meal. Chef's, Cobb, chicken Caesar, tuna, and taco salad: All of these fit the nutritional profile of the Whitaker Wellness Weight Loss Program. Plus they're easy to fix and widely available in restaurants. (Make sure you hold the croutons, tortilla chips, bread, and crackers.)

Here's a good thing to know about salad dressing. Acidic foods retard the emptying of food from the stomach, which slows the release of blood sugar. Vinegar, which contains acetic acid, has been shown to dramatically reduce the postprandial (after meal) blood sugar surge, improve insulin sensitivity, and help control weight. When volunteers drank two tablespoons of apple cider vinegar before two of their daily meals for four weeks, they lost an average of two pounds, and some lost up to four. Weight didn't budge in a control group. Carol Johnston, Ph.D., the Arizona State University professor of nutrition who conducted this study, speculated that vinegar may interfere with enzymes that break down carbohydrates, allowing them to pass through the digestive system without being absorbed. While you may not be inclined to drink vinegar as an aperitif, let Italian or oil and vinegar be your salad dressings of choice. (Or drink your water with a squeeze of lemon—the acids in lemon and lime juice likely have a similar effect.)[2]

If you're a sandwich junkie, you'll have to get a little creative because bread is off limits. Instead of a hamburger, enjoy a patty melt (ground turkey or lean beef with a slice of cheese melted over the top). Stuff your tuna salad in a tomato shell or an avocado. Scoop your taco fillings up in lettuce leaves, or wrap your sandwich fixings inside deli meats and cheese slices. Again, you may feel like you're missing something here, but focus instead on what you're gaining: calorie reduction, appetite control, and a slimmer body.

If you can't muster the time or energy to eat lunch, at least have a meal replacement drink or bar with the recommended grams of protein and carbohydrate. Do not make the mistake of skipping lunch altogether, or you're likely to be raiding the kitchen or break room at work for a mid-afternoon food fix.

DYNAMIC DINNERS

Dinnertime is the time of the day for most of us to socialize and enjoy a meal with family and friends. The protein and carbohydrate content of your evening meals will be similar to that of lunch and breakfast: 20 to 25 grams of protein and around 10 grams of carbohydrate. Select a three- or four-ounce serving of your favorite source of protein: chicken, turkey, fish, shrimp, lean meat, tofu. Spice it up with your preferred seasonings: teriyaki, Cajun, curry, garlic, Dijon. "Barbecue it, boil it, broil it, bake it, sauté it," to steal a phrase from *Forrest Gump's* Bubba Blue. Then, rather than partitioning your plate into the usual triangle of meat; vegetables; and potatoes, rice, pasta, or another starch, load up on vegetables.

You'll be surprised at how many vegetables you can eat and still stay within the 10-gram carbohydrate target. That's because plant foods contain a lot of water and a significant amount of fiber. Fiber is technically a carbohydrate, but since it is not absorbed as it passes through the digestive tract, you don't have to include it in your carbohydrate count. Subtract the grams of fiber from total grams of carbohydrate and you'll have the number of net, or available, carbs. A cup of most cooked vegetables (green beans, broccoli, Brussels sprouts, zucchini, squash, onions, kale, chard, turnip greens, spinach, and other leafy greens) gives you fewer than 10 grams of carbs. With raw vegetables you'd have to eat an entire head of romaine or iceberg lettuce, eight cups of spinach, two tomatoes or bell peppers, 10 stalks of celery, a whole cucumber to approach this level. (See Chapter 12 for charts of suggested serving sizes.)

If you're one of the surprisingly large number of Americans who say they don't like vegetables, perhaps it's because the last time you ate them they weren't prepared properly. Vegetables don't have to be bland or boring. Buy the freshest produce available (spend a little extra for organic if you can find it). Fresh spinach sautéed with a little garlic, for example, rises head and shoulders above frozen or, heaven forbid, canned spinach. And don't commit the common mistake of overcooking vegetables. Green beans and broccoli aren't supposed to be soggy and limp, but slightly firm and crunchy. You just might surprise yourself and discover that you actually like vegetables.

SUCCESSFUL SNACKING

In some circles, *snacking* is a naughty word. Not in mine. I believe any diet that does not include snacks is doomed to fail. If you're hungry between meals, you're going to eat, so why not build snacks into the plan? Snacking helps maintain a robust metabolism. Just as skipping meals or going on a very low-calorie diet signals your body to stop burning calories and store them as fat (that old survival tool for times of famine), snacking or eating more frequent small meals of the right types of food keeps your fat-burning mechanisms in gear.

Select your snacks carefully. Like your meals, they should contain some protein and lesser amounts of carbohydrates (seven or eight grams of protein and five or fewer grams of carbs). Suggested snacks include a quarter cup of nuts; a stalk of celery with peanut or almond butter or cream cheese; a quarter cup of cottage cheese with some chopped peppers or tomatoes; and a stick of string cheese or a hard-boiled or deviled egg with a few baby carrots, cherry tomatoes, or bell pepper rings. These may not be the world's most exciting snacks, but they will do exactly what they're intended to do: satisfy your hunger and tide you over until your next meal.

Another snack-time option is an appropriate-sized serving of a meal replacement drink. Measure out the equivalent of seven or eight grams of protein and five grams of carbohydrate (amounts will vary depending on the drink). Pure protein drinks can be jazzed up by blending in a quarter cup of berries or other fruit, unsweetened cocoa powder, or instant coffee sweetened with a little stevia or xylitol. (See below for more on these healthy sweeteners.)

In the three-week meal plan in Chapter 14, I've included two recommended snacks per day, in the mid-afternoon and in the evening after dinner. If you find you need a mid-morning snack, go for it. On the other hand, if you aren't hungry and don't feel like you want a snack, say, after dinner, don't force yourself to eat. You'll likely find as time goes by and your blood sugar swings even out, that snack time may eventually pass you by unnoticed.

"WHAT CAN I DRINK?"

Water should be your beverage of choice, and you should drink a lot of it—a minimum of eight and preferably 10 glasses of water daily. Water fills you up, which encourages you to eat less, but according to an intriguing German study reported in 2003, it also burns calories. Healthy, normal-weight volunteers were given two cups of water to drink, and within 10 minutes, their metabolic rate began to rev up. After 30 to 40 minutes it had increased by an average of 30 percent! The researchers who conducted this study estimated that 40 percent of this increase was due to the heating of the water from room temperature to body temperature while the remainder was attributed to an increase in fat and carbohydrate burning stimulated by the sympathetic nervous system. This suggests that the recommended eight cups of water will burn off a very significant 100 additional calories daily.[3]

This reminds me of a weight loss tip I heard a few years back from a physician I know in Oklahoma. He swears he lost 35 pounds simply by eating ice. When you eat ice, your body temperature falls, and to return to normal, your body has to generate energy—by burning calories. It takes 80 calories to heat two quarts of water from 32 degrees (freezing) to the normal body temperature of 98.6 degrees. However, it takes 240 calories to melt two quarts of ice cubes and then heat the water to 98.6 degrees. Although I confess I've never seen any research to support this novel method of weight loss, the math makes sense. Give it a try if you like, but don't break any teeth (dentists advise against chewing ice), and avoid "brain freeze."

Unlike many diets, alcohol is allowed on the Whitaker Wellness Weight Loss Program. A daily five-ounce glass of wine, an ounce of hard liquor mixed with water or soda, or a light beer is not going to blow your diet. In fact, study after study agrees that drinking moderate amounts does not lead to weight gain—and it is actually associated with weight loss in women. According to a large health survey conducted in England, women who consumed one to two drinks a day had a 15 percent lower BMI than those who did not drink.[4]

As I mentioned in Chapter 4, alcohol increases thermogenesis. The reasons for this are something of a mystery. The calories in pure alcohol come not from protein, fat, or carbohydrate but from ethanol, which contains about 65 calories per ounce. Although the human body can use ethanol for energy (it is first converted in the liver to acetate), it doesn't use it very efficiently. Therefore, it increases the metabolic rate by 10 to 30 percent, causing some calories to be burned rather than stored. Alcohol also favorably affects the cells' sensitivity to insulin and is linked with decreased insulin resistance, which is associated with obesity.

Let me make it clear that I am not suggesting you start drinking alcohol to lose weight. But if you enjoy a daily drink, there's no reason to stop. Be careful what you mix your spirits with: scotch and soda is one thing; rum and Coke is another. And note that beer does contain carbohydrates, so make it light beer and have a protein-rich snack such as an ounce of cheese along with it. Also remember that drinking reduces inhibition, which could make those chips and pretzels at the bar mighty hard to resist.

Caffeine is also acceptable on this program. I know some studies show that caffeine mobilizes blood sugar, which triggers a release of insulin that could overshoot the mark and make you hungry. But other studies demonstrate that it increases metabolic rate and burns calories. I am very familiar with both sides of this argument, and I'm firmly in the pro-caffeine camp. In my personal and professional experience, I've found caffeine to be an asset for people trying to lose weight.

Although many health experts are down on our favorite upper, coffee has a number of health benefits. It enhances cognitive performance, quickens reaction time, and promotes alertness and sustained attention. It restores flagging energy, can stop a migraine in its tracks, and relieves symptoms of asthma. It improves endurance so much that Olympic athletes can be disqualified for using high doses of caffeine. In addition, coffee is a good source of antioxidants. A 2005 study revealed Americans get more antioxidants from coffee than any other source![5]

I'm the first to admit that too much caffeine has a downside, including headaches, tremors, heart palpitations, and indigestion. However, I am convinced that moderate intake is a health plus. Anyway, since more than half of American adults drink coffee every day, I figure you're already experiencing enough deprivation on this diet, so I'm not going to take away your morning cuppa Joe (unless, of course, you simply can't resist having a doughnut or Danish along with your coffee).

An even better source of caffeine is green tea because, in addition to caffeine, it also contains epigallocatechin-3-gallate (EGCG). EGCG is a top dog in the polyphenol family of nutrients, which are known for their potent antioxidant activity. EGCG also promotes thermogenesis and fat burning. I personally make a point of drinking several cups of green tea daily. Remember, green tea isn't just for weight loss. It also protects against heart disease, diabetes, cancer, and a laundry list of other diseases.

I've already spoken my piece on fruit juice: Don't drink it. It contains too many calories and carbohydrates. The one and only exception is six to eight ounces of low-sodium tomato or V8 juice, which can be substituted for other carbohydrates in a meal or snack. I'm sure you know that sugar-laden sodas are off the menu, and so are diet sodas. As you'll see later, the safety of the artificial sweeteners in these drinks is highly speculative. Furthermore, a handful of studies suggest that high consumption of diet sodas and other foods made with artificial sweeteners may actually increase caloric intake and craving for sweets.

TAMING THE SWEET TOOTH

Speaking of sweets, if you'd as soon sacrifice a week's vacation as you would give up desserts, you don't just have a sweet tooth—you have a sweet fang.

The best way to conquer any addiction is to go cold turkey, and that's what you're doing on the Whitaker Wellness Weight Loss Program. Don't tease yourself with a bite of chocolate cake. It's just too darn easy to eat the whole thing. Once you've achieved your weight loss goal, you can have the occasional dessert. But if overeating of sweets and desserts has contributed to your weight problem, for now you need to just say no. (Remember the contract you made. Is that piece of pie really worth the money you'll have to give to your least favorite cause?)

As the mainstay of this program is whole, fresh foods, I'm not going to spend much time warning about all the hidden sugars in prepared foods. You're not going to be eating them anyway. Suffice it to say that, like salt, sugar in its many guises is added to so many different foods that you must pay close attention to food labels. Sucrose, dextrose, fructose, lactose, high-fructose corn syrup, honey, fruit juice, and maple, corn, rice, and barley malt syrups: All these sugars are concentrated carbohydrates that stimulate the release of blood sugar and insulin and should be avoided.

As I mentioned above, I do not recommend calorie-free artificial sweeteners such as acesulfame-K (Sunnett, Sweet One), saccharin (Sweet 'N Low), and especially aspartame (Nutrasweet, Equal, Spoonful). Aspartame, the world's most popular chemical sweetener, is broken down in the body into formaldehyde, methanol, and other toxins. It has been linked to dizziness, headaches, nausea, vision problems, and slurring of speech, symptoms so common that they are known as "aspartame disease." Although the industry-funded studies on aspartame passed safety tests with flying colors, independent research has revealed serious safety concerns. I strongly suggest that you avoid this artificial sweetener.

If you need to sweeten up your tea or yogurt, try stevia. This calorie-free herbal extract, which has a 1,500-plus-year history of use in South America, contains no carbohydrates and does not affect blood sugar levels, making it perfect for those trying to lose weight. Just a few drops of a liquid concentrate or a dusting of powdered stevia is all you need to lend sweetness to any food. It's the sweetener of choice at the Whitaker Wellness Institute.

Running a close second is xylitol, a natural sweetener that looks and tastes like sugar. Although xylitol is not calorie free, it is very slowly metabolized and has an extremely low glycemic index and load. It is what is referred to as a sugar alcohol, similar to mannitol and sorbitol, so its net or available carbohydrate count is inconsequential. The only reported side effect of xylitol is gastrointestinal distress if you eat too much.

If you feel like you have to use an artificial sweetener, go with sucralose (Splenda). It's made by chemically modifying a sugar molecule so your body cannot break it down and thus it passes through the gastrointestinal tract unabsorbed. As a result, it does not raise blood sugar or add calories. Sucralose has been under close scrutiny since it was first introduced in 1998. I've scoured the research on it and conclude that it is safe. I would still recommend stevia or xylitol first, but as far as I can tell, sucralose beats other artificial sweeteners hands down.

PORTION DISTORTION

I've heard the argument that oversized portions are the cause of our epidemic of obesity. Granted, eating more calories certainly contributes to weight gain, and Americans eat an average of 250 more calories a day than 25 years ago. But I firmly believe that if you eat the right foods, portion control will naturally follow. Of course, some people overeat when they're bored or stressed or simply in the habit of eating a lot. But most of you who are trying to lose weight are conscious of these triggers and are doing your best to avoid them. You overeat because you're hungry, and as I've explained in detail in earlier chapters, you're hungry because you're eating foods that initiate a physiological response that compels you to eat more.

On the Whitaker Wellness Weight Loss Program, you will be focusing on food composition, rather than portion control. You'll find it easy to eat less because your brain won't be screaming out every couple of hours telling you to refuel. Your next snack or meal won't be the main thing on your mind.

Throughout this chapter I've told you to aim for 20 to 25 grams of protein and 10 grams of carbohydrate per meal, because that translates into portion sizes that are more than adequate for most people. If you have a large frame or you engage in manual labor or otherwise burn up a lot of calories with physical activity, you may need to eat more. If you're petite or sedentary, you'll likely eat less. I want you to get up from the table completely satisfied. If you're still hungry, feel free to eat more lean protein and low-carbohydrate vegetables.

STAYING ON TRACK WHILE EATING OUT

I dine out a lot. Connie and I travel a fair amount for business and pleasure, but even when we're home, we're fortunate to live in an area where there are many great restaurants, and we like to eat out. We aren't alone. Sixty percent of Americans eat in restaurants at least once a week and 30 percent do so multiple times. Eating out can be a challenge. At home, nobody brings you a basket of fragrant, warm bread, and you don't have to look at plates of fettucini Alfredo or smell freshly baked brownies. In a restaurant, you may have to deal with the sight and smell of foods that are completely off limits, and it's crucial that you don't let these temptations blow you out of the water.

For starters, go in with the right frame of mind. There's something about eating in a restaurant that encourages us to let our guard down. We rationalize that we're good at home, so why shouldn't we treat ourselves when we're out? Look, if the only time you eat out is on your anniversary, I'd say order what you want. But if you eat out several times a week—or even more if you travel a lot—you've got to stop kidding yourself that this is a special occasion. It's not. It's everyday life.

It is very easy to adhere to the Whitaker Wellness Weight Loss Program in restaurants as long as you keep your contract in mind and follow a few basic guidelines. The first rule of dining out is to not walk into a restaurant famished. I know this sounds counterintuitive as you're going there to eat. But we've all had the experience of sitting down at a table and feeling so hungry that the bread or chips are gone before we even open the menu. If you've cut out starches and sugars, ravenous hunger is not likely to be an issue for you. If it is, simply eat a small, protein-rich snack—peanut butter and celery or a small handful of nuts—before you go out to take the edge off. If you're taking a bulk-forming, stomach-filling fiber supplement, take it before you leave home as well, along with a glass of water.

Next, select your restaurants carefully. If you're one of those people who can't smell pizza without devouring it, a pizza parlor is not your best bet. If the dish to die for in your favorite Chinese restaurant is egg rolls and orange chicken with lots of rice, better stay away from that one too. If you're a regular at the neighborhood café and they bring you a cinnamon roll for Sunday breakfast, no questions asked, there's another one you might pass on until you get the hang of this. The time will come when you can dine with friends and not have menu envy. In the meantime, make it easy on yourself by avoiding the restaurants that push your hot buttons.

When you sit down in a restaurant, get rid of obvious temptation. Turn down the obligatory basket of bread or chips. Order a beverage, preferably water, regular or sparkling, or iced tea, and drink a glassful. Now, open your menu. What you're looking for is fish, seafood, poultry, or lean meat; vegetables; and salad. Yeah, I know some of the other things on the menu are more appealing. It doesn't matter. You're going to order fish, seafood, poultry, or lean meat; vegetables; and salad.

Ask your waiter questions about the menu. If you don't know that chicken Florentine contains spinach and possibly cheese, ask. (It's a good choice.) If you're uncertain about chicken or veal Parmesan, find out. (It's breaded and off limits.) Find out how things are prepared. Baked, broiled, grilled, sautéed, stir-fried, poached, or steamed are good; breaded and deep fried are not so good. Try to ascertain what's in soups, sauces, and salad dressings. You're treading on thin ice when you order these things in restaurants because it's hard to know exactly what's in them. While the marinara sauce and cream of broccoli soup you make at home may be perfectly acceptable, you'd be surprised at how many cooks use sugar and flour as flavor enhancers and thickeners. If you do order sauces and dressings, order them on the side and eat them in moderation.

If the menu offers no perfect choice, ask for substitutions. Many entrées come with a starch such as potatoes or rice and a vegetable. Tell the waiter you'd like to replace the starch with extra vegetables or a green salad. Order the chicken sandwich without the bread or the stir-fried shrimp and vegetables without the rice. Eat your fajitas sans tortillas and your tacos and moo-shoo pork wrapped in lettuce leaves. In the rare event that there is nothing on the menu you can eat, invent something altogether.

One of my favorite things to order in restaurants is a piece of salmon on top of a big salad with oil and vinegar-based dressing; it's absolutely delicious. Another off-menu item I sometimes order for dinner is an omelet.

Nine times out of ten the chef will be happy to prepare what you request— it's not as if you're asking for anything very complicated. As a rule, nicer restaurants are more amenable to special requests than lower-priced ones. That's not to say you can't ever eat in fast-food joints. Just stick to salads and order your sandwiches minus the bread.

10 RULES FOR DINING OUT

1. Don't go into a restaurant famished. Eat a small protein-rich snack beforehand to take the edge off.

2. Stay away from restaurants that will sabotage your diet.

3. Send the basket of bread or tortilla chips away.

4. Ask questions about the menu and request substitutions.

5. Order a moderate-sized piece of fish, seafood, poultry, or lean meat; salad; and vegetables—no rice, potatoes, and other starches.

6. Ask for your protein selection to be grilled, broiled, baked, or sautéed, not breaded or fried.

7. Order salad dressing and sauces on the side.

8. Share an entrée, or eat half of your own and take the rest home in a doggie bag.

9. Drink lots of water or iced tea.

10. Say no to dessert.

Another thing you need to watch for in restaurants is serving sizes. They're simply out of control. In a sampling of foods from popular family-type, fast-food, and take-out restaurants, researchers from New York University found that servings of cookies, cooked pasta, muffins, steaks, and bagels were 700, 480, 333, 224, and 195 percent, respectively, larger than those recommended by the USDA and the Food and Drug Administration

(FDA). That's a whole lot of supersizing going on. Of course, you don't have to eat everything you're served, but whether it's a habit or a carryover from childhood ("Think about the starving children in Africa." "You can't leave the table until you've cleaned your plate."), we tend to eat what's put in front of us. So be conscious of portion sizes. Share an entrée with a friend, or ask for a carryout container and save half of your meal for the next day.[6]

We've covered a lot of ground in this chapter, and to make it easier for you to reference, I've arranged a lot of this material for easy accessibility in Chapter 12. Now, let's move on to another part of the Whitaker Wellness Weight Loss Program that sets it apart from others: specific strategies for curbing appetite and promoting fat burning.

7

HOW TO CURB YOUR
APPETITE AND EAT LESS

Have you ever felt so hungry you could eat a whole plate of cookies or a pint of ice cream in one sitting? Do you sometimes find it hard to eat just a handful of nuts or chips rather than the entire bag? Most of us who have to watch our weight have at one time or another been a slave to what William Shakespeare described as the "universal wolf"—appetite.

The desire to eat is a basic survival mechanism, and caving in is not simply a lack of willpower. When your body's biochemical signaling systems push hunger messages to the forefront of your brain, even Superman would have a hard time resisting. So don't get down on yourself. Stop blaming your lack of will and realize that hunger, rather than being your worst enemy, is nothing more than a primal reflex to keep you alive and well.

That said, I want to make it very clear that eating yourself silly is not what Mother Nature had in mind when this instinct was honed. What was once an asset—making sure we stored enough fat to carry us over through times of famine—is a liability in our environment of perpetual plenty. This is why, although I've touched on this concept throughout this book, I'm devoting an entire chapter to things you can do to control your appetite.

PROTEIN FILLS YOU UP,
STARCHES AND SUGARS FILL YOU OUT

Let's quickly review the chemistry of hunger. The hypothalamus is the area of the brain that regulates hunger and satiety. It receives feedback from leptin, ghrelin, and other hormones and messenger molecules that influence appetite and eating behavior. The hormone most central to the Whitaker Wellness Weight Loss Program is insulin: It's the one we know the most about and one you can control through diet.

As we discussed earlier, insulin is a nutritional storage hormone released in response to elevations in blood sugar. When you eat large amounts of fast-burning carbohydrates, you get a huge influx of blood sugar, and the pancreas must secrete large amounts of insulin to clear it out. In doing so, it often drives blood sugar too low. This causes the hypothalamus to sense that the brain is not getting enough fuel, so it turns up the volume on hunger signals—signals that, as you know, are almost impossible to ignore.

If you want to control your appetite, first and foremost you must stay away from starches and sugars. There's a French proverb that goes something like this: "Appetite comes with eating. The more one has, the more one would have." That's exactly what's going on when you eat starches and sugars. Even though you've just loaded up on calories and have plenty of stored fat, you find yourself, much to your dismay, eating once again. Cutting out the foods that wreak havoc with blood sugar and insulin will go a long way toward normalizing your body's complex biochemical signaling systems that govern appetite.

Second, eat more protein. Make sure you include a moderate serving of fish, seafood, poultry, egg whites, cottage cheese, soy, or other sources of lean protein with every meal and snack. Protein is highly satiating. It fills you up, tides you over, and puts an end to food cravings. It also discourages overeating. Numerous studies show that replacing some of the carbohydrates in the diet with protein results in a dramatic reduction in overall calorie intake—as much as 300 to 400 fewer calories in some cases—and leads to significant weight loss.

Break the painful cycle of blood sugar surges and crashes that promote binge eating once and for all by making these dietary changes a permanent part of your life.

FABULOUS FIBER

Eating more fiber will also put the brakes on appetite. Second to protein, high-fiber carbohydrates are the most satiating of all foods. In addition to providing bulk and filling up the stomach, fiber stimulates the release of cholecystokinin, a hormone secreted in the small intestine that signals satiety. It also slows the transit of food through the gastrointestinal tract, which retards the release of glucose and the spikes that can lead to low blood sugar.

Fiber significantly increases feelings of fullness and suppresses hunger pangs. In a study at the University of Texas Southwestern Medical Center, 12 men and one woman who were fed a high-fiber breakfast consumed less food at lunch than those who ate the same number of breakfast calories but no fiber. In fact, those eating a fiber-free breakfast ate as much at lunch as the study participants who had only water for breakfast.[1]

You can increase your fiber intake by eating more vegetables, fruit, nuts, seeds, and legumes and by taking supplements. Bulk-producing fiber supplements absorb water, expand, and fill up your stomach. Taking them before meals sends satiety signals to the brain and discourages you from overeating—and also reduces cholesterol, prevents constipation and hemorrhoids, and lowers blood sugar. The most popular type of supplemental fiber is psyllium (Metamucil); the ones we use at the clinic are glucomannan and ground flaxseed. (We'll return to these in Chapter 9 when we discuss nutritional supplements for weight loss.)

IN PRAISE OF SNACKING

If mealtime finds you ravenous and going back for seconds and thirds, between-meal snacks might be just what you need to control your appetite. My patients are sometimes surprised when I recommend snacking, but a small serving of protein-rich food in the mid-morning, mid-afternoon, and/or evening has been shown to not only take the edge off hunger but to trim the caloric content of meals. Eating smaller, more frequent meals (every three hours or so) also appears to accelerate metabolic rate. That's why we've built snacks into the Whitaker Wellness Weight Loss diet.

Make sure your snacks contain the right balance of protein and carbohydrates: about seven grams of protein and five of carbohydrate. A hard-boiled egg and some raw vegetables, celery with peanut butter, nuts, cottage cheese, deli meats and cheese—these snacks will tame your appetite, prevent overeating at meals, and promote weight loss.

KEEP A FOOD JOURNAL

When overweight patients tell me they eat like a bird but can't lose weight, I ask them to keep a food journal for three days. I suggest you give this a try. It forces you to step outside your normal eating routine and really become aware of what you eat. Simply write down every food and drink that passes your lips, how much you consume, and the time you eat.

This exercise can be quite illuminating. Many people underestimate their food intake. A cookie here, a double serving there, a soda or café mocha mid-afternoon: These "little" things can add up to enough calories to sink any weight loss goal. Some discover that the low-fat, high-carbohydrate foods they thought were good for them, such as whole grain pretzels, crackers, and other "health" foods, are actually undermining their weight loss efforts. Others realize they eat out of boredom or when they're stressed or upset. Keeping a food diary will help you ascertain what eating behaviors have contributed to your weight gain and provide insight as to how to correct them.

DRINK AWAY HUNGER

What has zero calories, costs nothing, and reins in your appetite? Water, of course. Water is one of the most powerful weight loss agents I know. Research shows that drinking lots of water suppresses hunger and, as we'll discuss in the next chapter, increases metabolic rate. So if you find yourself rooting around your kitchen for something to eat, drink a large glass of water and wait half an hour. This will likely hold you over until your next snack or meal. A tall glass of water 30 minutes before meals, perhaps with a fiber supplement, is also recommended.

Coffee and tea can put a lid on hunger as well. The caffeine in these beverages not only increases metabolic rate by virtue of its effects on the central nervous system, but it is also a mild appetite suppressant. My experience and that of my patients is that a nice hot cup of coffee or tea can get you through the mid-morning or mid-afternoon slump and tide you over until the next meal. Green tea's fat-fighting prowess goes beyond caffeine. It also contains epigallocatechin-3-gallate (EGCG), a polyphenol that revs up thermogenesis. When you feel the need to put something in your mouth, make it a sip of coffee or tea. Be aware that excess caffeine can cause stomach upset, insomnia, headaches, and palpitations. It may also interfere with sleep, so don't drink it late in the day.

GET ENOUGH SLEEP

I told you in Chapter 4 how sleep and weight problems are intertwined: Inadequate sleep increases the risk of obesity. Researchers from Columbia University found that obesity rates were 73 percent higher in people who slept no more than four hours per night and 23 percent higher in those who slept six hours, compared to people who got seven to eight hours of sleep. Why does sleep matter so much? Because sleep deprivation upsets the hormones that affect appetite and metabolism. Inadequate or poor quality sleep is associated with decreased levels of leptin and increased levels of grehlin, resulting in keener appetite and greater food intake. Poor sleep also hampers physical and mental performance, which puts the kibosh on motivation and exercise.[2]

Do not underestimate the importance of a good night's sleep for weight control and overall health. Establish a bedtime routine by going to bed at the same time each night. You should avoid caffeine after 3:00 in the afternoon (or earlier for some) and refrain from exercising within three hours of bedtime. To prevent waking up hungry in the middle of the night, eat a light protein-based snack before bedtime. If your sleep is disturbed by nighttime awakenings, learn stress reduction techniques that will help you go back to sleep. If you have trouble falling asleep, consider supplementing at bedtime with melatonin (1 to 3 milligrams), valerian root (300 to 500 milligrams), or 5-HTP (50 to 100 milligrams; more on this supplement later).

If you snore heavily and you're overweight, listen up. I used to snore at an Olympic-caliber volume. Although it affected everyone within a 25-yard radius, I wasn't losing any sleep over it—until I discovered that I had sleep apnea. Snoring is caused by the soft tissues in the back of your throat rattling around and partially blocking your airway. This blockage frequently becomes complete, and breathing stops altogether until oxygen deprivation arouses you enough to start breathing again. These episodes of breathing cessation are called sleep apnea. It is a very common condition that wreaks havoc with your sleep and upsets levels of appetite-regulating hormones, dramatically increasing the risk of obesity. Sleep apnea is also linked with diabetes, hypertension, stroke, and other serious diseases.

I now use a continuous positive airway pressure (CPAP) machine every night. It's a small mask worn over the nose attached to a device that gently blows pressurized air into the airway to prevent the soft tissues in the throat from collapsing. Thanks to this simple device, I sleep like a baby: no snoring, no tossing and turning, and no starting and snorting to catch my breath. If you suspect you may have this problem, talk to your doctor or contact the American Sleep Apnea Association at www.sleepapnea.org. Getting a handle on sleep apnea could make all the difference in the world in your weight and your overall health.

CONFRONT YOUR EMOTIONAL TRIGGERS

This chapter would not be complete without touching on emotional eating. If you've ever eaten in response to emotions rather than hunger, you know what I'm talking about. Eating for comfort is unbelievably common. You're bored, so you have nothing better to do than scrounge around for something to eat. You're depressed, and nothing makes you feel better than eating ice cream or another "comfort food." Anger, frustration, anxiety: All these emotions can trigger overeating.

We learned in childhood—actually in infancy—that food is soothing. It makes us feel good. Perhaps that's why many of the foods we turn to in times of stress are those that bring back positive memories. When researchers from the University of Illinois surveyed more than 1,000 consumers, they found that the favored comfort foods for women were ice cream, chocolate, and cookies; for men, they were ice cream, soup, and pizza or pasta. The reasons the people in this survey gave for selecting these foods were not because they tasted good but because of past associations and personality identification: Mom's homemade soup or the ice cream that was awarded as a special treat during childhood.[3]

Identifying the specific situations and feelings that trigger overeating is the first step in overcoming emotional eating. The second step is actually breaking the habit. Get out a pen and paper and make a list of alternatives to emotional eating. Read a book. Call a friend. Do a chore. Play with your children or your pet. Practice breathing exercises or deep relaxation techniques. Go for a walk. (Exercise is my favorite alternative because while it keeps you positively occupied, it also burns calories and makes you feel less hungry.) There is no end to the activities that will take your mind off eating. Copy your list and tape it to your refrigerator. The next time you feel like reaching for food when you're not really hungry, this list will stare you in the face. Over time, your emotional triggers will lose their power as substituting alternative behaviors becomes routine.

SUPPLEMENTS THAT TAKE THE EDGE OFF

I want to close this chapter by touching on nutritional supplements that take the edge off hunger and food cravings. Chapter 9 is entirely devoted to the supplements that help with weight loss, so I won't go into details here, but I do want to make you aware that your health food store has a plethora of safe, natural substances that can dramatically increase your odds of achieving your weight goals.

One of them is 5-hydroxytryptophan (5-HTP). When a patient comes to me complaining of carbohydrate cravings, especially if they are accompanied by depression or anxiety, I recommend this supplement. It works by increasing levels of serotonin, a neurotransmitter, or chemical messenger, in the brain that affects appetite, mood, and sleep. (As I mentioned above, it also helps you fall asleep.)

If a patient's weight is primarily in the abdominal area and he also has diabetes or hypertension, I suspect insulin resistance and recommend chromium and lipoic acid. These nutrients increase insulin sensitivity and also help with appetite control. EGCG from green tea; hydroxycitric acid

(HCA); glucomannan and flaxseed; and *hoodia gordonii*, an herbal extract from an African cactus, also help with weight control by reducing hunger.

I'll give you all the particulars about these supplements and more, including specific doses, in Chapter 9. But now, let's look at the other side of the weight loss coin: burning fat.

8

DON'T STORE FAT, BURN IT!

In my 30 years of counseling patients who are trying to lose weight, I've found that hunger and food cravings are far and away the most common reason people give up on diets—they just can't handle fighting the constant urge to eat. That's why the Whitaker Wellness Weight Loss diet works so well. It tames this very real physiological drive and makes passing up food easier than you can possibly imagine.

The second most common failure of weight loss programs I've seen over the years is that they don't produce results fast enough. We are a notoriously impatient culture. We want results and we want them now! If you've been discouraged by lack of progress on other weight loss plans, here's another thing you're going to love about the Whitaker Wellness Weight Loss Program: You will see results quickly. That's because, in addition to cutting appetite, this diet also stimulates the burning of fat. And that translates to weight loss.

Let's review what fat burning is all about. Right now, as you're sitting in your chair reading this book, you are burning calories. Inhalation and exhalation, the beating of your heart, and the myriad other biological processes that keep you alive use energy. The number of calories required at rest is your basal metabolic rate (BMR). Additional energy is expended by activity of any kind, by the muscles you use to keep you upright in your chair, by your digestive tract as you break down the food you've eaten, and by your physical movements as you go about your day. All these activities increase thermogenesis, or the production of heat in the body, and this requires energy.

The total amount of energy you expend in a day may be as little as 1,200 calories if you are sedentary, all the way to up 6,000 or more if you are exceptionally active. But whatever your metabolic rate happens to be, if you are overweight, your caloric intake surely exceeds your body's caloric expenditure. To lose weight, you must either eat fewer calories (which you're well on your way to doing) and/or burn more calories. Here are some tips on how to stop storing fat and start burning it.

IT'S ALL ABOUT EXERCISE

I've said it before, and I'll say it again: You can lose weight on the Whitaker Wellness Weight Loss Program if you don't exercise, but exercise will speed your weight loss and make it more enduring. That's because physical activity is the most effective means of burning calories. You'll use energy just sitting around playing with your kids (about 150 to 175 calories an hour). But if you go out and jog for an hour, you'll easily quadruple the number of calories burned. Walking, jogging, swimming, cycling, and other aerobic activities involving the continued, rhythmic use of the large muscles of the body make the heart pump faster, the lungs work harder, and burn calories.

The fact that aerobic exercise helps control weight is hardly earthshaking news. If you're reading this book, however, you may not have put it into practice. Everybody knows they should exercise regularly, yet only a small percentage actually do it. This book contains an entire chapter on exercise, and much of it is devoted to getting over the mental hump that seems to prevent most people from becoming physically active. In it, I share with you the motivational techniques that have helped thousands of my patients get started on an exercise program and, more important, stay on it. Exercise, especially when you are out of shape, can be painful, and it is human nature to avoid things that hurt. What you have to do is make the pain of *not* exercising outweigh the pain of exercising. To learn how to make a commitment to include this very important activity in your daily life once and for all, see Chapter 10.

BURN CALORIES IN YOUR SLEEP

The other type of exercise I focus on in Chapter 10 is anaerobic, or resistance, exercise. I've extolled the virtues of aerobic exercise for as long as I can remember. I was a jock in high school and college, and I've done some pretty significant aerobic exercise endeavors as an adult, including running seven marathons and riding a bicycle across the United States. However, I was a little slow on the uptake in my appreciation of resistance exercise. Now I know that it is every bit as important as aerobic exercise, especially if you're trying to lose weight.

Your basal metabolic rate, as we discussed above, is the amount of energy you use at rest. People who are naturally thin often have a higher than average BMR, meaning they burn more calories even when they're doing nothing. There is one proven way to increase your BMR: build more muscle. Muscle cells are loaded with mitochondria, the sites in the cells where energy is produced, and naturally burn more calories than fatty tissue. Anything you can do to increase your muscle mass will increase your BMR, so you'll burn more fat, even in your sleep. And there is one proven way to build more muscle: resistance exercise.

Chapter 10 includes a comprehensive resistance exercise routine that targets all of the major muscle groups, complete with detailed instructions. (For further instruction, these exercises are demonstrated on the Whitaker Wellness Weight Loss Program DVD, available at www.whitaker weightloss.com.) The best part of this routine is that it doesn't require a gym membership or special equipment, yet it is guaranteed to produce results. So when you're making your commitment to exercise, do not overlook the importance of strength training. It will make weight maintenance over the long haul much, much easier.

FOODS THAT TURN UP THE THERMOSTAT

The Whitaker Wellness Weight Loss Program is specifically designed to put your body into fat-burning mode. Glucose is your cells' preferred fuel, but when there is inadequate glucose in the bloodstream and the glycogen stores in your muscles and liver have been emptied, you quickly shift into your secondary energy system: fat burning.

That's why sugars, starches, and other sources of highly concentrated carbohydrates are not included in this diet. These foods drive up blood sugar and provide your cells with a constant source of glucose to use for energy.

When you exclude these rapidly absorbed carbohydrates and replace them with lean protein, healthy fats, and fiber-rich vegetables, your body has no choice but to start burning fat for energy.

Another reason protein is advantageous for those trying to lose weight is because it has a high rate of postprandial or diet-induced thermogenesis (DIT). This means it requires a significant amount of energy—20 to 30 percent of total calories—just to be digested and absorbed. Fat and carbohydrate, on the other hand, only require an energy utilization of 0 to 3 percent and 5 to 10 percent, respectively. So if you want to burn more fat, eat more protein. You'll burn up twice as many calories eating a high-protein/low-fat meal as you will a high-carbohydrate/low-fat meal.

Fish seems to be particularly effective at turning up the thermostat. Several studies have shown that people who eat lots of seafood have lower levels of leptin, a hormone that beefs up appetite and fat storage, and are less likely to be overweight.[1] It turns out that this may be because of the omega-3 fatty acids that are especially abundant in salmon, sardines, mackerel, tuna, and other cold-water, fatty fish. When these fats replace other fats in animal diets, there is decreased weight gain and accumulation of fat in the abdominal area, along with improved metabolism of fats and glucose.[2] I strongly advise you to include wild salmon and other omega-3-rich fish in your diet several times a week and to make fish oil capsules part of your daily nutritional supplement regimen.

Other fat-burners in your kitchen cupboards include cayenne, black pepper, ginger, and turmeric. These culinary spices not only turn on the flavor of food but also turn up your fat-burning mechanisms. While the effects of these foods are mild, they do increase thermogenesis. If you've ever broken into a sweat after eating hot peppers, you can understand this phenomenon. Peppers contain a compound called capsaicin, which is the best studied of these thermogenic spices. In addition to boosting metabolism, capsaicin has also been shown to suppress appetite. When Dutch researchers gave red pepper powder in tomato juice or capsules to study volunteers 30 minutes before meals, they reported increased satiety, and they ate less at mealtime. If you enjoy spicy food, I encourage you to use these herbs liberally.[3]

WET YOUR WHISTLE

I already mentioned the appetite-suppressing benefits of drinking water, but as you may recall from Chapter 6, it also increases thermogenesis. German researchers found that drinking two cups of water increased metabolic rate by 30 percent within 30 to 40 minutes. In addition to requiring energy to heat water up to body temperature, drinking water also arouses the sympathetic nervous system, which further increases metabolic rate. They concluded that eight cups of water a day would increase caloric expenditure by 100 calories—about as much as you'd burn swimming for 20 minutes![4]

There may be some added advantage to drinking your water cold. I mentioned a friend of mine who lost a significant amount of weight by eating ice. Although I am unaware of any research showing that ice or cold drinks actually result in weight loss, it makes a lot of sense, as they would burn up even more calories heating up to body temperature. Whether you prefer your water iced or at room temperature, there are many, many good reasons to drink eight to 10 glasses of water every day, whether you're trying to lose weight or not.

Unless you have a problem with alcohol, I see no reason not to enjoy a glass a day of wine, light beer, or spirits. In fact, it may actually ratchet your metabolic rate up a notch. Like protein, alcohol has a high diet-induced thermogenic rate of 10 to 30 percent. This means that when you drink an ounce of ethanol (the form of calories in alcohol), you burn up to 30 percent of those calories metabolizing it. Alcohol also has positive effects on insulin sensitivity. The bulk of the studies on alcohol and weight do not support a link between moderate intake of alcohol and weight gain. In fact, moderate alcohol intake is associated with a reduced BMI in women.

The bottom line is that a drink a day will not sabotage your weight loss program and may even facilitate it. If you are a drinker, limit yourself to one light beer, five-ounce glass of wine, or one-ounce shot of hard liquor. (Do not use fruit juice or soft drinks as mixers.) Be very aware that even one drink is enough to cloud judgment in some people and make staying on the straight and narrow all the more difficult. Drink time is also synonymous with munchie time, so if alcohol makes it difficult for you to pass on the bar snacks, avoid it altogether. And make sure you balance your drink with an ounce of cheese or another protein-rich snack.

COFFEE, TEA, OR EGCG

Caffeine is a well-known thermogenic agent that, in addition to increasing metabolism, also cuts appetite. I have always maintained that caffeine, from either coffee or tea, is an excellent diet aid. In a 2005 study published in *Obesity Research,* Dutch researchers followed 76 overweight or moderately obese men and women during a four-week low-calorie diet and for three additional months to observe weight maintenance. They found that the study volunteers who drank lots of caffeine lost more weight and had less body fat and smaller waist circumferences than those with a low caffeine intake. The women in the study with high caffeine consumption also had reduced levels of leptin. The study concluded, "High caffeine intake was associated with weight loss through thermogenesis and fat oxidation [fat burning] and with suppressed leptin in women."[5]

For most Americans, caffeine means coffee, but an even better source of caffeine might be tea, especially green tea. Green tea is nature's most abundant source of epigallocatechin-3-gallate (EGCG), a polyphenol with very powerful antioxidant activity. EGCG is a hot commodity in medical research theses days and is being studied for the prevention and treatment of cancer, heart disease, diabetes, dental cavities, and many other conditions. In addition to these medicinal benefits, EGCG also simulates thermogenesis, so when you drink green tea, you get the cumulative fat-burning benefits of caffeine and EGCG. While black tea also has many health benefits, it doesn't contain the EGCG levels that green tea does, so if you're looking for a weight loss boost, stick with green tea.

Let me restate my warning that too much caffeine is not a good thing. It can overstimulate the nervous system and make you feel wired, shaky, and nervous. It can also increase heart rate, upset your stomach, and give you a headache. Moderate intake, however, is an overall health plus. In addition to improving mental and physical performance, it is associated with reduced risk of diabetes, Parkinson's disease, gallstones, and colon cancer. A cup or two of coffee or tea to start off your day or during a break at work makes you feel more alert, cuts your appetite, and turns up your fat-burning mechanisms. Do not, however, drink colas for their caffeine content. As we have discussed in previous chapters, the artificial sweeteners in diet drinks and the enormous amount of sugar in regular sodas are strictly off limits. If you feel jittery or otherwise uncomfortable when you consume caffeine, then it's not for you. Try some of the other fat-burners discussed in this chapter instead.

CAN CALCIUM PROMOTE FAT LOSS?

It has been observed in numerous scientific studies that people with high calcium intake are less likely to be obese than those who get little calcium in their diet. Back in the 1980s, scientists looking at the effects of calcium on hypertension observed that when study subjects ate more dietary calcium, their weight, along with their blood pressure, went down. We now know why: Calcium deficiencies promote fat storage. Low levels of calcium stimulate the release of hormones that help conserve calcium. At the same time, one of these hormones, called calcitriol, triggers fat storage and slows down fat burning.

The likely reason for this, according to Michael Zemel, Ph.D., of the University of Tennessee, is that the body equates low calcium levels with scarcity of food, so in addition to conserving calcium, these hormones also hang onto fat. Dr. Zemel conducted a study in which three groups of people ate the same low-calorie diet with differing amounts of calcium for six months. Those who got 400 to 500 milligrams of calcium per day lost an average of 15 pounds; those getting 800 milligrams lost 19 pounds; and those getting 1,200 milligrams (primarily from dairy products) lost 24 pounds and a higher percentage of body fat and abdominal fat.[6]

To sum this up, if you aren't getting enough calcium in your diet, you may have a tendency to gain weight even if you're doing everything else right. Considering that almost three-quarters of American adults do not get adequate calcium—they average only 400 to 500 milligrams per day—this could certainly be a factor in our epidemic of obesity. The Whitaker Wellness Weight Loss Program includes lots of reduced-fat cheese and cottage cheese to boost calcium levels and recommends 1,000 milligrams of supplemental calcium daily. While calcium supplements are not as well studied as dietary calcium in weight loss, they're an excellent way to hedge your bets and ensure adequate calcium intake.

SUPPLEMENTS TO INCREASE THERMOGENESIS

In the next chapter, we will take an in-depth look at nutritional supplements that increase fat burning. These include EGCG, caffeine, fish oil, and calcium, which we've already discussed, as well as extracts from bitter orange and ephedra.

Targeted nutritional supplements are an overlooked yet extremely valuable component of a weight loss program, especially during the dog days of a diet when you hit a wall or reach a plateau. Read on to learn more.

9

LOSE WEIGHT FASTER WITH NUTRITIONAL SUPPLEMENTS

The history of the weight loss industry is littered with "miracle drugs" once launched with great fanfare, only to be pulled from the market when their dangerous side effects were discovered. You probably remember fen-phen, the enormously popular drug duo (fenfluramine and phentermine) promoted as the end-all for curbing appetite and speeding weight loss. Skyrocketing sales came to a screeching halt in 1997 when researchers at the Mayo Clinic reported that a number of previously healthy patients developed serious cardiac valve problems while taking these drugs, and the drugs were subsequently removed from the market.[1]

Phenylpropanolamine (PPA) is another diet drug that bit the dust due to its adverse side effects. Marketed as an over-the-counter appetite suppressant and decongestant for more than 60 years, PPA was linked to an increased risk of hemorrhagic stroke (brain bleeding) and taken off the shelves in 2000. Researchers at Yale University School of Medicine found in a five-year study that this drug dramatically increased risk of disabling or fatal stroke. In fact, it was deemed responsible for up to 500 preventable strokes per year![2]

Today's top diet drugs are Xenical (orlistat) and Meridia (sibutramine). Xenical is a fat blocker that works by inhibiting the actions of lipase, an enzyme that digests fat, allowing about 30 percent of dietary fat to pass through the body unabsorbed. And while it's true that this drug does aid weight loss, it also causes gastrointestinal problems and embarrassing oily spotting. The biggest problem I see with Xenical is that you lose more than just weight—you also lose valuable fat-soluble nutrients such as vitamins A, D, E, K, beta-carotene and other carotenoids, and coenzyme Q10. This can lead to nutritional deficiencies, which likely explains why Xenical has such a long list of side effects.

Meridia is an appetite suppressant that increases brain levels of serotonin, a neurotransmitter that affects appetite, mood, and sleep. I'm leery of drugs that alter serotonin levels. This is the same neurotransmitter targeted by Prozac, Zoloft, Paxil, and other antidepressants. These selective serotonin reuptake inhibitors (SSRIs) have a very serious slate of adverse effects. They are required to carry a "black box" label (the most serious type of drug warning) stating that they increase suicide risk in children and teenagers, and the FDA has also issued a public health advisory warning of "the possibility of an increased risk for suicidal behavior in adults." Although the adverse psychiatric effects of Meridia may not be as severe as those of antidepressants, I would steer clear of this drug. Documented side effects of Meridia include elevations in blood pressure and heart rate, liver problems, headache, dry mouth, insomnia, and constipation.

I can understand why people who are frustrated in their weight loss attempts are looking for additional help, but drugs are not the answer. If you need an extra boost in addition to the Whitaker Wellness Weight Loss Program diet and exercise plan, your best bet is to skip the drugs and try targeted nutritional supplements.

WHY YOU SHOULD TAKE A MULTIVITAMIN AND MINERAL SUPPLEMENT

You may not think of your daily multivitamin and mineral as a weight loss supplement, and in the strictest sense of the word, it isn't. However, a good daily multinutrient supplement offers protection against obesity. Deficiencies of some nutrients are associated with weight gain, and despite the fact that we eat more calories than ever before, nutritional deficits are surprisingly common among Americans.

According to 2005 statistics from the USDA, 93 percent of Americans fail to get enough vitamin E, three-quarters get insufficient calcium, 56 percent get inadequate magnesium, and a third to a half of us have inadequate intake of vitamin C, vitamin A, and iodine. Now do you understand why I place such importance on vitamin and mineral supplements? Even if you think you're eating a good diet, you might not be getting enough of these basic nutrients, and that can have broad negative ramifications on your health.[3]

Nutritional deficiencies both promote and accelerate heart disease, dementia, hypertension, arthritis, osteoporosis, diabetic complications, vision loss, and, of course, obesity. In the previous chapter, I told you how calcium deficiencies are linked with increased risk of obesity. When calcium levels are low, hormones released to safeguard meager calcium stores also suppress fat burning and promote fat storage. Increasing your calcium intake by taking supplemental calcium is a powerful, yet overlooked tool for weight loss.

Iodine is a mineral required for thyroid hormone production, and thyroid hormones, as we discussed in Chapter 4, are a primary regulator of metabolism. Average iodine levels in this country have fallen 50 percent in the past 30 years, and during that time we have seen huge increases in thyroid disorders and obesity. We screen all overweight patients who come to the Whitaker Wellness Institute for thyroid function, and if it is low, we treat them with natural thyroid replacement. But to give your thyroid a fighting chance, it is crucial that you get enough iodine.

Even antioxidants, which are best known for protecting against free radical damage, may play a role in weight maintenance. Vitamin C levels are inversely related to body mass—the fatter you are, the lower your vitamin C levels, in most cases. People with adequate vitamin C level have been shown to burn 30 percent more fat during exercise than individuals with low vitamin C status. This means as simple a step as taking vitamin C supplements may make weight loss easier.[4]

Antioxidants also protect against the free radicals produced during exercise, which makes them all the more important if you're on the Whitaker Wellness Weight Loss Program. Researchers from the Antioxidant Research Laboratory of Tufts University have demonstrated that taking high doses of vitamin E lowers the exercise-induced production of free radicals. Vitamin E has also been shown to reduce muscle damage that occurs with weight training and to lessen morning-after stiffness and soreness.[5]

Other basic vitamins and minerals play a role in metabolism and energy expenditure, and when your cells do not have access to the nutrients they need, systems falter. Here are the doses of vitamins and minerals I recommend.

Nutrients	Effects on Weight Loss	Daily Amount
VITAMIN A	Antioxidant support.	3,500 IU
BETA-CAROTENE and mixed carotenoids	Antioxidant support.	16,500 IU
VITAMIN B1 (thiamine)	Energy production.	50 mg
VITAMIN B2 (riboflavin)	Energy production.	50 mg
VITAMIN B3 (niacinamide, niacin)	Energy production and blood sugar regulation.	100 mg
VITAMIN B5 (pantothenic acid)	Adrenal function and stress reduction.	50 mg
BIOTIN	Insulin sensitivity.	300 mcg
VITAMIN B6	Mood, energy, and gene expression.	75 mg
VITAMIN B12	Mood, energy, and gene expression.	150 mcg
FOLIC ACID	Mood, energy, and gene expression.	800 mcg
VITAMIN C	Antioxidant support and fat burning.	1,000 mg
CITRUS BIOFLAVONOIDS	Improved bioavailability of vitamin C.	150 mg
VITAMIN D (cholecalciferol)	Calcium absorption and metabolism.	800 IU
VITAMIN E (d-alpha-, gamma-, delta-tocopheryls, tocotrientols)	Antioxidant support.	400 IU
ALPHA LIPOIC ACID	Insulin sensitivity and appetite control.	200-400 mg
CHOLINE	Brain function and fat metabolism.	200 mg
INOSITOL	Mood and insulin sensitivity.	40 mg
CALCIUM	Fat burning.	1,000 mg
MAGNESIUM	Energy production.	500 mg
IODINE	Thyroid function.	150 mcg
ZINC	Insulin production.	30 mg
COPPER	Nervous system function.	2 mg
CHROMIUM	Insulin sensitivity and appetite control.	400-600 mcg
SELENIUM	Thyroid function.	200 mcg
MOLYBDENUM	Metabolism.	130 mcg

Do not be alarmed by what may appear to be "megadoses." The paltry doses of many nutrients recommended by the government are just not enough. I've been using large doses of vitamins and minerals in my practice for close to 30 years, and thousands of scientific studies show that they are safe and highly therapeutic. Unfortunately, you will not find these levels of nutrients in a one-a-day multivitamin. You'll have to spend a little extra to get a brand that contains higher doses, but, in my opinion, it's worth it.

I also recommend that all of my patients take two fish oil capsules as part of their basic daily supplement regimen. The omega-3 fatty acids in fish oil confer a host of health benefits, from dampening inflammation to reducing risk of cardiovascular disease to boosting mood—all of which are of particular concern if you're struggling with weight. Furthermore, fish oil has been shown to improve fat and glucose metabolism, yet another reason to include it in your daily supplement routine. Look for a fish oil supplement guaranteed to be free of lipid peroxides, mercury, and other contaminants, and aim for a minimum of 320 milligrams daily of both eicosapentaenoic acid (EPA) and docosahexaenoic acid (DHA), the most important omega-3 fatty acids.

Both multivitamins and fish oil supplements are safe and well tolerated. Very high amounts of vitamin C and magnesium cause gastrointestinal upset in some people, but this rarely happens in the doses noted in the chart on page 94.

ZEROING IN ON XANTHINES AND OTHER STIMULANTS

The most highly advertised weight loss supplements contain central nervous system stimulants that increase your metabolic rate, raise your body temperature (thermogenesis), and burn calories. Until the FDA yanked ephedra off the market (more on ephedra later in this chapter), it was dieters' favorite thermogenic agent. Now, supplement manufacturers depend on other ingredients to achieve the same end.

Chief among them are xanthines. You are no stranger to these exotic-sounding substances. The caffeine in your morning coffee or tea is the most widely used xanthine in the world; others include theophylline and theobromine. Xanthines have a number of medicinal uses. Theophylline is a common ingredient in asthma drugs, and caffeine is used in over-the-counter analgesics such as Excedrin as well as in drugs to increase alertness, such as No-Doz and Vivarin. Because of the thermogenic properties of caffeine and other xanthines, you'll also find them in many weight loss supplements.

Another popular stimulant in weight loss supplements is *Citrus aurantium* (bitter orange). Bitter orange contains synephrine, a chemical cousin of ephedrine, which also elevates metabolic rate but appears to have less of an effect on the cardiovascular system. At least five studies have shown that this supplement promotes thermogenesis and weight loss. Harry Preuss, M.D., of Georgetown University Medical Center, stated in an article in the *Journal of Medicine*, "*Citrus aurantium* may be the best thermogenic substitute for ephedra."[6]

AN ELEGY FOR EPHEDRA

The best-studied, most effective weight loss supplement is ephedra, or ma huang (*Ephedra sinica*). This herb has been used in China for at least 5,000 years, and its active ingredients, ephedrine alkaloids, have been used in Western medicine for the treatment of allergies, asthma, and obesity. It is such an effective bronchodilator, meaning it relaxes and enlarges the bronchioles to allow easier breathing, that a synthetic version, pseudo-ephedrine is the active ingredient in many popular cold, sinus, and asthma remedies.

Scores of clinical studies have shown ephedra to be an effective therapy for weight loss because it revs up metabolism and increases fat-burning, particularly when used in combination with caffeine. In fact, this combo has been demonstrated in multiple studies to be as effective as any prescription weight loss drug.[7]

I'll be the first to agree that ephedra may also have other not-so-positive effects. Because it is a central nervous system stimulant, it arouses the sympathetic nervous system, which controls the body's fight-or-flight response and may raise blood pressure and heart rate, alter heart rhythm, and cause anxiety and insomnia in some people. It can also cause a nervous, edgy feeling that leaves you irritable and crabby. Ephedra should obviously be used with caution and should not be taken by people with significant diseases or those taking certain prescription and over-the-counter drugs. But it's important to note that these warnings are identical to those of dozens of popular remedies people use every day.

That's why it's unconscionable that in 2004 the FDA banned ephedra, claiming it was a health threat that could trigger anxiety, hypertension, heart attacks, strokes, and more. This is a shame, since ephedra is one of the few proven therapies for weight loss— and a farce since there are more than 100 over-the-counter drugs that contain a synthetic form of ephedra. If anything should be banned, it's some of the prescription drugs that kill more than 106,000 Americans and harm millions each and every year. Ephedra's dangers pale in comparison to theirs.

In May 2005, a federal judge in Utah overturned the FDA's blanket ban on ephedra, citing that the FDA could provide no evidence showing that ephedra at doses of 10 milligrams or lower posed any health risk. If and when ephedra returns to the market, the recommended dose is 10 milligrams one to three times a day.

One man who benefited from bitter orange is Gerhard, who had good success on the Whitaker Wellness Weight Loss Program but desperately wanted to slim down before attending his class reunion. When he was two months and 15 pounds away from his goal, he hit a brick wall—the scale simply would not budge. Try as he might, he was stuck. As it turned out, bitter orange was the key that got him past this plateau, and last April he showed up at his reunion in tiptop shape.

Xanthines are decent weight loss agents in their own right, and they are often found in combination with bitter orange and other ingredients in weight loss supplements. If the product label mentions guarana, cola nut, tea, yerba mate, or cocoa, count on it containing caffeine and other xanthines. Bitter orange is sometimes listed as *Citrus aurantium* or synephrine. The usual doses are 100 to 200 milligrams each of caffeine or other xanthines and bitter orange, one to three times a day between meals.

I urge you to use caution with this class of weight loss supplements. Do not use them if you are pregnant or if you have high blood pressure, irregular heart beat, anxiety, or another serious medical condition. Furthermore, some people do not tolerate stimulants and even small amounts make them wired. If you notice any jitteriness, nervousness, heart palpitations, increased anxiety, or other adverse symptoms, discontinue them at once. However, most people can handle the recommended amounts of these thermogenic agents just fine. Used judiciously, they can jump-start a weight loss program or, as they did for Gerhard, shift it into a higher gear.

GREEN TEA: WEIGHT LOSS ELIXIR

Green tea extract is one of the best supplements for dieters because it contains two of nature's most effective weight loss aids, caffeine and epigallocatechin-3-gallate (EGCG). As you know, caffeine revs up thermogenesis. But green tea's star ingredient is EGCG. EGCG is a catechin, a member of the larger family of plant compounds called polyphenols, and it is something of a wonder nutrient. First and foremost, it is an incredibly potent antioxidant. Cancer, heart disease, infections, Parkinson's disease: EGCG has been shown to protect against all these and more. But EGCG is also a unique weight loss aid because it tackles weight on two fronts—fat burning and appetite suppression.

The effects of EGCG, especially when used in combination with caffeine, have been studied for more than a decade now. In one of the more recent studies of this potent duo, Canadian researchers gave study volunteers capsules containing 200 milligrams of caffeine and variable doses of EGCG three times a day 30 minutes before meals. Compared with placebo, daily energy expenditure increased by an average of 180 calories in the volunteers taking EGCG and caffeine.[8]

For maximum fat-burning effect, look for a standardized EGCG extract or a green tea extract with a specified concentration of EGCG. Take as directed; doses vary according to EGCG concentration. It may be taken alone or in combination with caffeine or other weight loss supplements. EGCG is exceptionally safe, and there are no contraindications to its use.

CUT CARB CRAVINGS WITH 5-HTP

When I ask my patients to give up the starches and sugars that have caused their weight gain, they often express doubts about their ability to comply, citing out-of-control carbohydrate cravings. But once they get started on the diet, these cravings vanish. That's because the Whitaker Wellness Weight Loss Program puts an end to the blood sugar swings that make you feel hungry all the time.

There is a nutritional supplement that also helps control carbohydrate cravings: 5-hydroxytryptophan (5-HTP). 5-HTP is an amino acid derivative that is a direct precursor to serotonin. Serotonin is best known for its effects on mood, but it also helps regulate appetite. Unfortunately, serotonin imbalances are quite common, especially in people who have been on a high-carbohydrate, low-protein diet—such a diet is often deficient in the amino acids required for the synthesis of serotonin. Unlike Prozac and other SSRI antidepressants, 5-HTP does not block normal serotonin metabolism; it simply provides the body with the requisite building blocks to produce adequate levels of this important neurotransmitter. Therefore, it is much, much safer and has none of the adverse effects of the antidepressants.

If you have food cravings, particularly for bread, pasta, and other carbohydrates, consider trying 5-HTP. It has been shown in clinical studies to reduce appetite, cut carbohydrate cravings, and assist in weight loss. (As an added bonus, it also relieves depression and insomnia.) The suggested dose is 50 to 100 milligrams one to three times a day, taken between meals. Look for a natural 5-HTP extracted from Griffonia seeds. Do not take this supplement if you are taking any kind of perscription antidepressant, tramodol, caridopa, or a triptin drug. Large doses can cause nausea or diarrhea; otherwise, 5-HTP is safe and well tolerated.

FIGHT FAT WITH FAT

If your big belly is getting your down, conjugated linoleic acid (CLA) might be your supplement of choice. This naturally occurring fat, found in meat and dairy products, helps normalize levels of leptin and resistin, hormones that regulate appetite, fat storage, and insulin sensitivity. It has been shown to be particularly effective at increasing muscle mass at the same time it promotes fat loss. In a 2004 study conducted in Norway, 180 overweight men and women were randomly assigned to take CLA or a placebo (olive oil) for one year. Over that time, the study subjects taking CLA lost an average of 7 percent more body fat and gained almost 2 percent more lean body mass than those taking olive oil.[9]

CLA seems to target visceral adipose tissue (VAT) and preferentially decrease abdominal fat. This is good news on several fronts because VAT is linked with insulin resistance and increased risk of diabetes and cardiovascular disease. CLA is also under investigation as a natural therapy to both prevent and retard the growth of several types of cancer, including breast, prostate, colorectal, lung, skin, and stomach.

If you decide to give CLA a try, select your supplement carefully. University of Nebraska researchers found that only the 10-12 isomer of CLA promotes fat loss and breakdown. The best-studied CLA supplement is Tonalin, and the recommended dose is three grams per day (one gram with each meal). Mild gastrointestinal symptoms have been reported with large doses of CLA, but most people tolerate it fine. Although some studies have reported that CLA improves insulin sensitivity, a couple of small studies found that it may worsen blood sugar control, so people with diabetes should monitor their blood sugars when taking this supplement.[10]

DHEA BUSTS BELLY FAT

Another supplement that might help deflate your belly fat, particularly if you're in your forties or older, is dehydroepiandrosterone (DHEA). DHEA is a hormone produced by the adrenal glands that is the precursor to estrogen, testosterone, and other hormones. Levels in the blood peak around age 20, then fall as we age. Hundreds of studies link declines in DHEA levels with a number of age-related health problems, including abdominal obesity and metabolic syndrome.

Researchers at the Washington University School of Medicine in St. Louis enrolled 52 older men and women who had low blood levels of DHEA-sulfate (a blood maker of DHEA status) and were overweight and inactive. They determined their levels of abdominal fat by magnetic resonance imaging (MRI), then gave them either 50 milligrams of DHEA or a placebo daily at bedtime. Repeat MRIs after six months revealed that the visceral abdominal fat in the women taking DHEA decreased by 10.2 percent and in the men by 7.4 percent. Subcutaneous abdominal fat was reduced by approximately 6 percent in both genders. DHEA also improved insulin sensitivity, leading the researchers to conclude: "DHEA replacement therapy might reduce the accumulation of abdominal fat and protect against development of the metabolic/insulin resistance syndrome."[11]

I've been using this over-the-counter hormone with my patients for more than 20 years. Numerous studies have shown that in addition to fighting fat, DHEA also reduces symptoms of lupus and, in older people, boosts mood and memory, heightens libido and sexual function, improves sense of well-being, and increases bone density.

DHEA is not for everyone, but if you are 45 or older, I suggest getting a DHEA-sulfate blood test to determine if your levels of this hormone are low. If they are, give supplemental DHEA a try. Our usual starting dose is 25 milligrams daily for women and 50 milligrams for men. Have another blood test three to six months after starting on DHEA to make sure the dose you're taking is keeping your blood level of DHEA-sulfate in the targeted range (the normal levels for a young adult). Because DHEA is converted into testosterone, excessive amounts can cause acne or promote facial hair growth in women. These side effects will clear up as soon as the dose is cut back or discontinued. I do not recommend DHEA for patients with breast, ovarian, or prostate cancer.

A DHEA derivative, 7-keto-DHEA, is used in weight loss supplements because it's supposed to stimulate thermogenesis, possibly by increasing the activity of thyroid hormones. While I don't use it in my clinic, I'm keeping my eye on 7-keto-DHEA, especially for people younger than 45. In one small study, volunteers taking 100 milligrams twice a day in combination with exercise and diet lost twice as much body fat as a group taking a placebo.

FILL UP WITH FIBER

We've discussed the importance of fiber in weight loss, and I told you how high-fiber foods provoke the release of cholecystokinin in the small intestine. This hormone signals the hunger center in the brain that you're full, which is one reason why high-fiber foods are so satiating. Because Americans as a rule do not get adequate fiber in their diet, I strongly recommend supplemental fiber for many reasons, including weight loss.

My favorite fiber supplements are flaxseed and glucomannan, derived from the konjac root native to Asia. When you stir stir these fiber sources into water, they immediately begin to thicken, and when you drink them, they form a thick, gelatinous mass in your stomach that fills you up. Supplemental fiber also slows the absorption of carbohydrates and thus has a positive effect on blood sugar and insulin levels.

Several clinical studies have shown that fiber promotes weight loss and adherence to diet. In one double-blind study of glucomannan, obese patients who took glucomannan with water before meals lost an average of five and a half pounds in eight weeks—without exercising more or going on a diet. Glucomannan, flaxseed, and other fiber supplements also relieve constipation, lower cholesterol, and help with blood sugar control.[12]

The suggested dose of glucomannan is half a teaspoon mixed in an eight-ounce glass of water 30 minutes to an hour before meals. (Avoid glucomannan capsules, because they could potentially stick in and block the esophagus.) For flaxseed, its three tablespoons, ground and mixed in water. (It may also be sprinkled on salads and other foods.) Supplemental fiber is safe and well tolerated, although it can cause gas and bloating. To minimize this, build up to the suggested dose slowly.

CHROMIUM AND ALPHA LIPOIC ACID
IMPROVE INSULIN SENSITIVITY

Because insulin resistance figures so heavily in our epidemic of obesity, I want to tell you about a couple of nutritional supplements that will increase your cells' sensitivity to insulin and also help with weight loss.

Chromium is a trace mineral that helps control appetite by signaling the hypothalamus, the brain's hunger center, that it's time to stop eating. Even more important is chromium's role in glucose metabolism: It facilitates the action of insulin and the uptake of glucose into the cells. People with type 2 diabetes and insulin resistance (think abdominal fat) reap particular benefits from this mineral, as it has been shown to lower blood sugar and improve glucose control. In a 2004 review, British researchers pooled all the studies on the effects of chromium on weight loss and found it to have modest but observable effects.[13]

Deficiencies in this mineral are quite common in the United States, likely because of our high consumption of refined grains, which are stripped of natural chromium content and may even promote chromium loss. The best supplemental sources are chromium picolinate and chromium polynicotinate, and the suggested dose is 200 micrograms two to three times daily with meals. Some studies indicate that chromium may become toxic in amounts over 1,500 micrograms per day, so do not exceed the recommended dose.

Alpha lipoic acid may also facilitate weight loss. We know that this potent antioxidant improves insulin sensitivity, and it is a well-accepted therapy for diabetes and diabetic complications. But animal studies demonstrate that it also suppresses appetite by activating satiety signals in the brain that lead to reduced food intake. It appears to increase energy expenditure as well. High-dose lipoic acid (several hundred milligrams per day) is currently being tested as a potential weight loss drug.[14]

It is premature to prescribe very high doses of lipoic acid for weight loss. However, I strongly recommend 100 to 200 milligrams twice a day for overweight people with diabetes or other signs of insulin resistance. Individuals with diabetes should monitor blood sugar levels because it can drive them downward, and medication dosages may need to be lowered. (This is a good thing.) Although exceptionally high intakes may cause gastrointestinal upset, lipoic acid is safe and generally very well tolerated.

WHAT ELSE IS OUT THERE?

Walk into your health food store and peruse the weight loss and body-building supplement sections. You'll be amazed at what's out there. I want to give you an overview of additional weight loss supplements—the good and the bad.

Chitosan is a fiber extract taken from the outer skeletons of crabs and other crustaceans. It is supposed to bind to fats in the intestines and shuttle them out of the body. The "fat-trapping" effects of chitosan aren't what they're cracked up to be. Even if this supplement did work, I wouldn't recommend it, because it would also soak up fat-soluble nutrients just as the drug Xenical does. Save your money on this one.

Garcinia cambogia is extracted from a fruit native to southern India. Its active ingredient, hydroxycitric acid (HCA), has both thermogenic and appetite-suppressing effects. It inhibits the conversion of glucose to fat and influences glycogen formation in the liver. Because full glycogen stores signal the brain that you're full, HCA makes you feel less hungry, so you naturally eat less. In one study, obese patients taking Garcinia cambogia extract with chromium lost an average of 11.4 pounds in eight weeks, while a placebo group lost just four pounds. Other studies, however, have been a wash. I'd consider this a second-string supplement, but if you want to try it, take 250 milligrams of HCA three times a day with meals. Because Garcinia cambogia is eaten as a food in India, it has a very good safety profile.

Hoodia gordonii, a succulent native to southern Africa, is used by San Bushmen in the Kalahari Desert to stave off hunger and thirst during long treks. It contains a compound called P57 that stimulates the hunger/satiety area of the hypothalamus and "tricks" the brain into thinking you're full. When P57 is administered to animals, they eat 40 to 60 percent less food than they usually eat. Preliminary human studies demonstrate that hoodia is highly effective in reducing appetite. In one study, obese people taking hoodia extracts ate 1,000 fewer calories than a control group taking a placebo—they just didn't feel hungry.

There is concern that many of the hoodia products on the market are mislabeled and do not actually contain hoodia, or they have too little of the herb to have a therapeutic effect. The dose that appears to be effective is 3,000 to 4,000 milligrams of a powder made from the plant's stems and roots; a concentrated extract, of course, would require a lower dose. I think hoodia is very promising and, as far as I can tell from the little research done on it to date, safe. If you decide to try hoodia, purchase it only from a reputable manufacturer.

Phaseolus vulgaris, which is derived from white kidney beans, is touted as a starch blocker. An earlier version of this supplement was pulled from the market during the 1980s due to safety concerns. The newer version is supposed to be safer and reportedly works by deactivating amylase, the enzyme required for starch digestion and absorption. While some of the initial studies of *Phaseolus vulgaris* are compelling, undigested carbohydrates in the large intestine is not a good thing. I'll have to wait for more research before I feel comfortable recommending any starch blocker.

Pyruvate is a naturally occurring compound that is required in the production of ATP, the fuel produced in the mitochondria that runs your cells. While very large doses of pyruvate (a minimum of 20 grams per day) have been shown to result in weight loss, the usual recommended dose is just 3,000 to 5,000 milligrams. Pyruvate might be a reasonable adjunct to other weight loss aids, but I'm not convinced that these lower doses on their own are that helpful.

SO WHAT DO I TAKE?

We've talked about a lot of different supplements in this chapter, and I've summed up their actions, doses, and safety information in the appendix. Yet you may still be asking the question, "What do I take?"

I can only tell you what I do with my patients. Rather than focusing on a single herb or ingredient, I prefer a broader approach when it comes to weight loss supplements. The one I recommend most often at my clinic contains thermogenic caffeine from green tea, appetite-suppressing and fat-burning EGCG, and insulin-sensitizing chromium and lipoic acid. When used in concert with a multivitamin and mineral supplement—and, of course, a good diet and exercise program—it has helped many patients jump-start a program or get over a discouraging plateau in their weight loss efforts.

Beyond that, I simply address my patients' individual needs. If someone is having carbohydrate cravings, I suggest 5-HTP. If it's bothersome belly fat, I recommend DHEA for those over age 45 and CLA for younger people. If a patient has metabolic syndrome or other signs of insulin resistance, I suggest chromium and lipoic acid. None of these supplements are mutually exclusive—they can safely be taken in combination, depending on your individual needs.

I want to reiterate that nutritional supplements that curb appetite and increase thermogenesis are not the centerfold of the Whitaker Wellness Weight Loss Program. However, they are a valuable, yet overlooked, tool in taming America's epidemic of obesity.

10

EXERCISE: THE ULTIMATE FAT-BURNER

Let me warn you up front: This chapter is not going to tell you anything you haven't already been told about the many benefits of exercise.

You already know you cannot sustain normal weight without regular exercise. You already know that fad diets, prescription weight loss drugs, and magic supplements that promise to melt away pounds with no changes in your lifestyle are absolute bunk. You already know that if you eat more calories than you burn, you'll gain weight, and if you burn more calories than you eat, you'll lose weight—and that the best way to burn more calories is to exercise.

You know that if you exercise, you increase your lean muscle mass and shed excess body fat, causing your resting metabolic rate to increase and your body to burn more calories even when you're sleeping. You know that carrying around extra pounds puts you on the fast track to type 2 diabetes, hypertension, cardiovascular disease, stroke, gallbladder disease, respiratory dysfunction, gout, osteoarthritis, certain types of cancers, and even premature death.

You and everybody else in this country, including the two-thirds of adults who are overweight and the one-third of overweight adults who are obese, have known this for some time, so the incentive is obviously there to get up and get moving. Yet fewer than two out of 10 adults exercise regularly, and three out of 10 get almost no physical activity. We use our cars for 93 percent of all trips and log a mere 1.4 miles per week of walking. It's not enough, not by a long shot.

You know that exercise is the best prescription for a thinner body and better health, but it's not lack of knowing that's the problem—it's lack of *doing*. Many of you, I am certain, have begun exercise programs with all the best intentions, only to slack off and eventually abandon them. What you lacked wasn't the knowledge that exercise is good for you. What you lacked was an incentive. So what you are going to learn in this chapter that *is* new is the most important key to successful exercise: consistency.

THE PAIN INCENTIVE

Exercise is a pain. No one, or at least very few, wakes up in the morning smiling and saying, "Wow! Now I can get on that treadmill!" In my opinion, those who do are deranged. Therefore, you need to devise a way to force yourself to do what you don't want to do. It's really quite simple: You make the pain of *not exercising* substantially greater than the pain of dragging yourself out of bed and exercising. And here is the way to do it.

First, as I described in Chapter 2, make a public contract with yourself. Write out what type of exercise you are going to engage in regularly. Whether you decide to bicycle, run, swim, or walk is not relevant. Choose any activity or combination of activities, but commit to it. Remember, you will be pledging to do a specific *behavior* (walking a mile a day or swimming 10 laps each morning) rather than the desired *result* (losing weight, fitting into a size 10). That's because the only thing you can completely control is your behavior.

That's just the first step. Next, spell out the consequences you will incur if you fail to fulfill your end of the exercise bargain. This consequence must be significantly more agonizing than the pain you're going to endure staying on the program. It might be that you promise to make out a check for $1,000 to your least-loved organization or to shingle your annoying uncle's roof. Just make sure that coughing up that money or nailing shingles in the heat of summer is substantially less appealing than the pain of staying on your exercise program.

Third, make this contract *public* to as many people as you can. Give them a copy of your contract. Ask them to check up on your progress. If you've got two people who are watching your progress, that will not give you nearly as much incentive as 20 people knowing what you're supposed to be doing and making sure you're doing it.

This kind of contract works only if you're honest. If you're not honest, don't waste your time. Go back and sit in front of the TV. People break contracts all the time but only if there are no consequences to pay. Even if you were tired this morning, you got up and went to work. If you hadn't, there would likely have been severe consequences. Constant incentives are the key to maintaining any kind of behavior. There's no mystery here. If you want to change a behavior, ramp up the consequences, and you'll increase your compliance and chances of success.

SILENCING THE EXCUSES

If you're taking the idea of this contract with yourself as seriously as I hope you are, you're probably running through all sorts of excuses for why you can't make the commitment to exercise.

But since permanent weight maintenance is highly unlikely without regular exercise, it's time to throw away the excuses.

NO TIME

Trying to fit exercise into your busy day may seem almost impossible, but it takes less time than you think. All you need to do to begin is to participate in some form of moderate exercise at least 30 minutes a day. That's it! Replace half an hour of TV with any type of physical activity and you're there. For a person weighing 154 pounds, walking can burn 280 calories per hour, and bicycling eats up 590. Even gardening or taking a short hike can work off an average of 350 calories per hour.

Look, we're all busy. That's why it's important to take the time to schedule exercise into your busy days. Whether you wake up half an hour early, fit some activity into your lunch hour, or skip one TV sitcom this evening, don't tell me you can't find 30 minutes to devote to your health and well-being.

TOO TIRED

Fatigue is a poor excuse to avoid exercise. The more sedentary you are, the less energy you'll have. You need to expend energy to get energy. Physical activity increases your oomph by strengthening your heart, lungs, and blood vessels. With regular, sustained exercise, your heart pumps more blood. With each beat, your lungs supply more oxygen and your arteries deliver more blood to your tissues. The end result is a body that does more work with less effort—and that means more endurance and energy for you.

Second, exercise acts directly on the brain to relieve depression, anxiety, and stress, all of which drain your energy. Exercise accomplishes this mood elevation magic largely via its ability to promote the release of endorphins. Endorphins, the brain's "feel-good" neurotransmitters, are naturally occurring chemicals that have an opiate-like effect in the body. Endorphin production begins after about 20 minutes of brisk activity and continues for hours thereafter. People who exercise regularly benefit from a natural and energetic high throughout the day.

TOO OLD OR SICK

Feeling old before your time? Nothing can make you feel younger—and maintain your independence—than regular exercise. And it's never too late to start. Researchers from Tufts University started a group of men and women in their 80s and 90s on a strength-training program. These were not your typical weightlifters—they were quite frail and most of them used walkers. Yet after 10 weeks, their muscle strength more than doubled, their gait was faster and steadier, and some of them were able to discard their walkers![1]

What about illness? A friend of mine with multiple sclerosis was deteriorating fast until she got a personal trainer and started on an intensive exercise program. A year later, she had no signs or symptoms of the disease.

Age and illness are not good excuses for avoiding exercise. In fact, if anything, they should be an incentive to become physically active.

GETTING STARTED

Both aerobic and anaerobic exercise are required to achieve and maintain a healthy body weight. Fast walking, jogging, swimming, cycling, and other fast-paced aerobic activities shift your heart and lungs out of first gear. They burn calories, condition your cardiovascular system, and increase insulin sensitivity. I strongly recommend aerobic exercise at least three days a week for a minimum of 30 minutes at a stretch. (For a great 30-minute aerobic workout, see the Whitaker Wellness Weight Loss Program DVD.) Whatever aerobic activity you choose, work out to the point where you get your heart rate up and you're breathing hard. If you feel like you're not working hard enough, you probably aren't.

Ideally, you want to reach your *training heart rate* and maintain it for a minimum of 20 minutes. To determine your training heart rate (in beats per minute), you first need to calculate your maximum heart rate. Subtract your current age from 220. If you are 35 years old, your maximum heart rate is 185; if you are 55 it is 165. You should never allow your heart rate to go above this number. Your training heart rate should be 75 to 85 percent of the maximum. For example, if you are 35 years old, 75 to 85 percent of the 185 maximum (185 x .75 = 139; 185 x .85 = 157) is 139 to 157. Therefore, you should aim for a pulse rate between 139 and 157 beats per minute.

To measure your heart rate while you're working out, find a pulse point at the inside of your wrist below the thumb or on your neck, count the number of times your heart beats in six seconds, and add a zero.

Anaerobic exercise, which is equally if not more important for weight control, targets certain muscle groups with resistance in order to increase the strength, tone, and size of your muscles. Each time you lift weights, your muscle fibers tear slightly. As they heal, they become stronger—this is how you build muscle. The more muscle you have, the higher your metabolic rate, and the more calories you will burn at rest, making it easier to maintain your ideal weight.

If you're a rookie at resistance training, the best way to begin is to get some instruction. It doesn't have to be with a personal trainer, although this is a very good option. A group class at your gym, some instruction from a friend experienced in weight training, or an exercise video that teaches proper technique would also work. I've provided some very explicit instructions for resistance exercises at the end of this chapter that you can do at home, and there's a Whitaker Wellness Weight Loss Program DVD that demonstrates them as well. Once you understand the basics and get the hang of it, you can continue on your own. If you commit to just two days of strength training a week you're doing yourself a tremendous service. Three days a week are even better, with a day of rest in between so your muscles have time to rest and rebuild.

If you are over the age of 40 or have a history of heart disease, hypertension, diabetes, irregular heartbeat, chest pain, shortness of breath, or pain in your legs or joints when walking, you should obtain medical clearance before you begin exercising. An exercise stress test is also advisable, for it allows your physician to pinpoint any potential problems you might have during exercise. Beyond that, all it takes is some hard thinking (making a commitment to yourself is serious business), planning, and ultimately just doing it.

1. MAKE A CONTRACT WITH YOURSELF

Make a commitment contract similar to the ones we discussed in Chapter 2. (A sample is included at the end of this chapter, or you can visit www.whitaker weightloss.com to print out a copy.) Decide on a very specific exercise behavior, such as walking for 30 minutes four days a week, going to the gym every other day, or doing a resistance exercise routine at home three days a week. Remember that you are pledging to change your behavior, not some nebulous outcome such as having bigger muscles or losing 20 pounds. It's fine to shoot for those goals, but what you're committing to is a specific exercise activity. Be very realistic. Do not commit to something you're not willing or able to do.

Tell your family and friends that you're going to start a new exercise program and there will be unpleasant consequences if you slack off. Ask them to keep an eye on you and even better, get someone to exercise with you. Having an exercise partner will make you more accountable, plus you'll be offering that person a chance to improve his or her health.

Here are a couple of sample contracts. Fred, a USC alumnus and huge football fan, pledged, "I agree to jog for 45 minutes every Monday, Wednesday, Friday, and Saturday and lift weights every Tuesday and Thursday for the next three weeks. If I so much as miss one of these scheduled sessions, I will give $500 to the UCLA football boosters club." Amanda set a lesser but adequate goal. "I agree to walk every other day for three weeks. If I so much as skip one day, I agree to give $50 to whoever runs against the incumbent in the next school board election."

2. PLAN YOUR EXERCISE SESSIONS

Before day one of your program, sit down with your calendar or a copy of the Weekly Exercise Log (also at the end of this chapter and at www.whitaker weightloss.com) and plan your exercise for the first week. Fill in the type and duration of the exercise and what days you'll be doing it. Carefully select a time of day to set aside for this activity: before breakfast, after you drop the kids off at school, after dinner, etc.

Once your weekly schedule is in place, all that remains is your follow-through. Post your forms, along with your commitment contract, on your fridge or in another prominent place. They will be a constant reminder of your personal commitment to improving your health and will keep you focused on what you need to do and when you need to do it.

At the end of the week, get out a new log sheet or calendar page and plan out the next week. In time, exercise will become a habit, just like flossing your teeth. It may never become your favorite thing in the world, but it will be part of your daily routine.

STAYING MOTIVATED

I'm 61 years old, and I've been extremely active my entire life. I participated in three sports in high school—football, basketball, and track—and was on the football team for two years in college. I've played tennis, squash, racquetball, and handball most of my adult life. In my 30s and early 40s I jogged regularly and ran seven marathons, including the Boston Marathon, as well as dozens of 10-kilometer races. I began biking in my late 40s and rode a bicycle across the country, covering over 3,500 miles in 10 weeks.

However, as I approached 60, I was burned out. Somewhere along the line I lost the motivation to exercise. I wasn't able to run as fast or jump as high. My knees took a pounding when I jogged, and I was slower on the court. So I looked into other types of exercise. For a year, I was into swimming. Four or five days a week I would trek to my health club and swim three-quarters of a mile (1,200 yards). I liked it because it was easier on my joints—swimming is ideal for people with arthritis, musculoskeletal injuries, or other physical problems—and it uses every muscle in the body. But after a while, I got tired of driving to the club, and I started to slack off. So I switched gears.

Today I work out at home on a treadmill and a Bowflex machine. A treadmill, in my opinion, is the best aerobic exercise machine there is because it doesn't slow down when you get tired. Bicycles and stair steppers allow you to slack off, but treadmills don't give you a break. The fancier ones can monitor your pulse, and if the machine determines you are working outside the target heart rate for your age and weight, it will slow down. It won't, however, ease up because you're lazy or bored.

As my exercise history illustrates, it's unlikely that you'll stick with one form of exercise your entire life. When you get tired of one activity, take up another. If you can't stand the thought of doing anything at all, try some of the suggestions below for getting active and staying motivated.

Get distracted. Exercise can be mind-numbingly boring. To get around this, create a distraction. The reason you see joggers wearing headphones is because music takes their mind off the task at hand. My wife works out on a stair stepper, and she's constantly reading while she's on it—she says it's the only thing that makes it tolerable. The form of distraction that works best for me is movies on DVD. It's hard to read on a treadmill. I almost killed myself when I flew off the back of the darn thing while trying to read. TV would be perfect, except there's no guarantee that what's on will hold your interest. That's why I prefer movies while I exercise. I've strapped a portable DVD player onto my treadmill so that it covers up the time and distance display. I pop in a movie, put in the earphones, push play, and I'm off. As I become engrossed in *The Mask of Zorro* or *Shrek* or *The Incredibles,* I work up a sweat and my heart gets pumping. But rather than focusing on the work of exercise, I'm into my movie. I often find that when I stop and look at the time, I've been exercising for 45 minutes without even realizing it. If I don't finish a movie, I find myself actually looking forward to exercising again so I can see the end. (Part of my bargain with myself is that I can only watch DVDs while I'm exercising.)

Make it social. When you make exercise commitments that involve other people, you'll exercise far more regularly. Get a walking or jogging partner and meet at a designated time several days a week. Organize a softball or basketball team among your coworkers and join the city league. Or get a group of friends together, plan a special activity such as a challenging nature hike, and train together for the event. You will be surprised at how fast you put on your walking shoes when someone's waiting for you at your front door.

Join a fitness program or class. Sports clubs and gyms of all kinds are everywhere. Walk in and ask about trial offers. Most gyms and fitness groups will let you try them out for a small fee or even for free. Take a fitness trial tour of your town and find out what it has to offer. Community centers also offer a multitude of seasonal sports activities for kids and adults from bowling to swimming to yoga. (I used to think yoga meant stretching until my stepdaughter put me through her paces, and I discovered that yoga can be a real aerobic and anaerobic workout.) Tennis, racquetball, and squash clubs have challenge ladders that require you to play regularly and compete against people of similar ability. Cycling clubs have weekly group rides, and running clubs organize regular jogs. Merely signing up for such activities forces you to work them into your schedule. If you join a group or class, particularly if you pay for it, you are likely to attend.

Sign up for personal exercise feats. Register for a walk-a-thon, 10-kilometer run, or marathon. Sign on for a long, scenic bike trip. Plan a hike into the Grand Canyon. Raise money for a worthy cause by getting donations and participating in a 5K walk some organizations hold yearly—and plan to beat the pants off the friends you finagle into joining you. Whatever goal you set, big or small, that upcoming date on the calendar will help motivate you to train before the big event.

Make exercise a part of your commute. Instead of driving to work every day, walk, if possible. Or try taking the bus or train. The walk to and from the station or stop will guarantee that you'll get some exercise daily, plus you'll save on gas. Another option is to get a bicycle and bike to the office. Once I had a routine where I drove my car, with bicycle strapped on a rack on top, for five miles of my 15-mile commute. Once I got off the freeway, I parked the car, jumped on my bike, and pedaled the remaining 10 miles. At the end of the day it was 10 miles back to the car, or I didn't get home!

Get more active in your daily regimen. If you are unwilling to commit to an exercise routine, at least make a point of becoming more active during the course of your day. Research suggests that making a conscious effort to fit in 30 minutes of physical activity during the day may be as effective as doing aerobic exercise in supervised classes several times a week. In a study published in the *Journal of the American Medical Association*, 116 men and 119 women aged 35 to 60 were randomly assigned to either a "lifestyle" activity group or a structured exercise class. After two years, participants in both groups were noted to have similar improvements in cardiopulmonary fitness, blood pressure, and percentage of body fat. Increase your activity by taking the stairs rather than the elevator. Select a remote parking space and walk to your destination. Use the extra 15 minutes before an appointment to take a walk around the office complex. Bound up the stairs two at a time, rake leaves, shovel the driveway, mow the grass, or vacuum vigorously. Accumulating 30 minutes of activity during the day isn't that difficult.[2]

Track your mileage with a pedometer. A great way to track your additional activity is with a pedometer, a small, inexpensive gadget sold in sporting goods and electronics stores. You simply clip it on your belt, and it counts the number of steps you take. We give pedometers to the patients who come to Whitaker Wellness and encourage them to walk the half mile between the clinic and the hotel where they stay. (We reward the person who clocks up the most steps in a week.) Pedometers have been shown to be very effective in increasing activity level and lowering blood pressure, blood sugar, waist girth, and weight. Aim for 10,000 steps a day.

DON'T FORGET TO STRETCH

Regardless of what type of exercise you engage in, each session should begin with five or 10 minutes of gentle stretching and warm-up to loosen your muscles and prevent strain and injury. Each stretch should be done slowly and held for 15 to 30 seconds. Never force a muscle or bounce during a stretch. When the muscle is stretched too far, it reacts by tightening slightly to protect itself from tearing, and you wind up with a muscle that is tighter than it was before you began the stretch.

Side Stretch: Stand up straight with your feet shoulder-width apart.

Keeping your right arm straight, extend it straight up over your head, fingers pointing to the sky. Keeping your body squared and your arm straight, gently lean to the left. Hold for 30 seconds. Repeat with the left arm.

Neck Stretches: From a sitting or standing position with your shoulders relaxed and your face forward, slowly tilt your head to the left, bring your ear towards your shoulder. Hold for 15 seconds, then bring your head to center and slowly tilt towards your right shoulder, holding for 15 seconds. Next, tilt your head again towards your left shoulder, then bend your neck and slowly roll your head across your chest until it is tilted towards your right shoulder. Roll back towards the left, and repeat. Finally, turn your head as far as you comfortably can to the left, as if you were trying to look behind you. Hold for 15 seconds, then repeat on the right side.

Shoulder Stretch: Stand up straight with your feet shoulder-width apart. Slowly roll your shoulders backwards through 10 large, exaggerated, complete circles. Then roll them forwards 10 times.

Thigh Stretch: Stand up near a chair or wall and put all your weight on your left leg. Bend your right knee to lift your foot behind you, reach back, and grasp your ankle with your right hand. (Hold onto the chair or wall to help maintain your balance.) Make sure you keep your lower back straight to avoid strain, and pull upward on the ankle until you feel a stretch in your thigh. Hold for 30 seconds. Switch legs and repeat.

Calf and Hamstring Stretch: Stand with your feet shoulder-width apart. Bring your left foot forward about 12 inches and flex your left ankle, toes pointing towards the ceiling. With a straight back, bend forward at the hips until you feel a stretch in your calf and hamstring. (Place your hands on your thighs to support your lower back.) Hold for 30 seconds, then repeat with the right leg.

Spinal Stretch: Stand up straight with your feet shoulder-width apart and place your hands on your thighs. Bend forward at your hips, letting your arms relax towards the floor. Now, very slowly, roll up to standing, one vertebrae at a time. Repeat three times.

Chest and Arm Stretch: Stand up straight with your arms at your sides and your feet shoulder-width apart. Extend both arms behind your back and clasp your hands together. To increase the stretch, raise your clasped hands a few inches. Hold for 30 seconds, then release.

In addition to warming you up for exercise, these stretches feel unbelievably good. Whenever you need a break from your desk or daily activities, try one or two of these stretches. They'll relieve the kinks in your neck and back, improve circulation, give your brain a needed rest, and actually increase productivity.

WHITAKER WELLNESS WEIGHT LOSS PROGRAM
AT-HOME RESISTANCE EXERCISE ROUTINE

Here's a muscle-building routine anyone can do at home. It requires no special equipment because it simply uses the weight of your own body as resistance. Before you begin, warm up with a stretching routine or a five- to 10-minute walk. Loose, warm muscles will respond better to the exertion of lifting weights with less chance of injury. Proper execution of these exercises is important to avoid injury and gain maximum benefits, so follow the descriptions carefully, or watch the Whitaker Wellness Weight Loss Program DVD. You should be able to do this routine in 20 or 30 minutes. It's best to rest a day between sessions, but you can do aerobic activities on the days you aren't strength training.

UPPER BODY

Pushups: Lie on the floor face down, hands shoulder-width apart. Keeping your stomach muscles tight, your back straight, and your toes on the floor, slowly straighten your arms and raise your body off the floor, then lower yourself back down to the starting position. (If this is too difficult, do a modified pushup with your knees on the floor.) Do as many pushups as you can in one minute, rest, then repeat.

Extended Arm Circles: Stand up with your feet shoulder-width apart and raise your arms out to your sides. With your elbows and wrists straight, make small, clockwise circles, about a foot in diameter, with your hands for 30 seconds. Reverse directions, and make counterclockwise circles for another 30 seconds. Relax and repeat.

Wall Pushups: Stand facing a wall, about an inch or two more than arm's length away. Without locking your elbows, extend your arms straight toward the wall at shoulder level and rest your palms against the wall, supporting your weight as you lean forward. Now lower your chest toward the wall, using only the strength of your arms to do so. Push back to the original position, again using only the strength of your arms. Repeat for a total of 15 repetitions. Rest, and repeat.

Biceps Curls: Stand with your feet shoulder-width apart and your arms at your sides. Bend your right arm at the elbow until your right hand is parallel to the ground, palm up. Place your left hand on top of your open palm. With your elbow tucked into the side of your waist and while pressing with your left hand to create as much resistance as you can handle, move your right forearm up so the hand is near your right shoulder, then move it straight down towards the right thigh. Do 15 repetitions, then switch sides. Rest and repeat.

CORE

Crunches: Lie on your back, legs bent at knees, feet flat on the floor, hands clasped behind and supporting your neck, elbows out. Without arching your back, slowly raise your shoulder blades off the floor. Hold for two seconds, concentrating on the tension in your abdominals. Lower yourself back down. Do 15 repetitions. Relax and repeat.

Bridge: Lie on your back with your knees bent, feet flat on the floor, and arms at your sides, palms facing down. Slowly lift your pelvis up so that your hips and lower back are off the floor, while your upper back and shoulders remain in place. Hold for five seconds, then slowly lower your hips back down to the floor. Relax and repeat 10 times. Rest, then do another set of 10.

LOWER BODY

Lunges: Stand with your feet together, hands on hips (near a wall or chair for balance, if needed). Step back with your right leg, and position yourself so your left knee is bent at a 90-degree angle directly over your left ankle and your thigh is parallel to the floor. Your right leg may be slightly flexed for balance. Hold for a few seconds, then return to standing and repeat with the right leg. Repeat 10 times on each leg, alternating sides. Rest and perform another set.

Quad Strengtheners: Sit in a chair with your back straight and buttocks tucked against the back of the chair. Place a towel under your knees for support, if desired. Slowly lift your left foot until the leg is horizontal in front of you. Hold for five seconds, then slowly lower your foot to the floor. Repeat with the right leg. Alternating legs, do 10 repetitions with each leg. Relax and repeat.

Step-Ups: Stand at the bottom of a set of stairs. With your toes facing forward, place your right foot on the first step. (If this isn't enough of a challenge for you, place your foot on the second step.) Holding onto the handrail, slowly step up onto the stair, straightening your right leg. (More advanced exercisers: With a straight knee, lift your left leg behind you.) Pause, then step back down to the floor. Repeat 10 times with the right leg and 10 times with the left leg for one set. Rest and complete a second set of 10 repetitions with each leg.

Squats: Stand in front of a chair with your feet slightly more than shoulder-width apart. Lean forward at the hips and, holding onto the chair if needed for balance, slowly lower your hips until you reach a near-sitting position. Pause, then slowly return to a standing position. Repeat 10 times. Rest, then do a second set of 10 repetitions.

Calf Raises: Stand up straight near a wall or chair. Slowly raise yourself up on your tiptoes as high as you can (steadying yourself with the wall or chair if you need to), pause for three or four seconds, and slowly lower yourself back down. Pause, then repeat 15 times. Relax for a minute and do another set. You can make this exercise more difficult by holding a weight in one hand, performing the movement more slowly, or rising on one leg at a time.

Flutter Kicks: Lie flat on your stomach, elbows bent, and your palms open on the floor near your shoulders. Breathing steadily, tighten the muscles in your buttocks and, keeping your legs straight, flutter kick your legs as if you were swimming. Continue moving your legs up and down for about 30 seconds, then relax. Repeat this sequence for a total of three sets.

WHITAKER WELLNESS WEIGHT LOSS PROGRAM
EXERCISE LOG

Date	Time & Duration	Activity
Sun.		
Mon.		
Tues.		
Wed.		
Thurs.		
Fri.		
Sat.		

COMMITMENT CONTRACT

I,_____ agree to _____

for three weeks beginning _____. If I so much as

_____

I agree to give $_____ to _____

Signed _____

Witnessed by _____ Date _____

You can visit www.whitakerweightloss.com to download these forms and sign up for e-mail reminders and exercise tips.

11

CONNECTING THE DOTS

I didn't write this book so it would gather dust on the shelf with all your other diet books. Getting down to your ideal weight—and staying there for the rest of your life—is not an impossible dream. The Whitaker Wellness Weight Loss Program is a connect-the-dots program that leaves nothing to chance. If you can follow directions and color between the lines, you will succeed. Let's review what is required of you.

1. MAKE A COMMITMENT TO CHANGE YOUR BEHAVIOR

I'm not going to reiterate the many adverse health and social ramifications of obesity. They will not inspire you to lose weight—if they did, you'd have slimmed down years ago. Awareness that a poor diet and inactivity have caused your weight problem is also no guarantee of successful weight loss. Nor is a nagging spouse, concerned friends, or a stern physician admonishing you to mend your ways. Knowing exactly what changes you need to make helps, but knowledge is not the same as action.

The missing ingredient is your personal commitment to make the specific changes in your day-to-day behavior that will result in weight loss. Giant steps, baby steps, one behavior, or the whole program—it's your call. Just make sure it's something you're willing to follow through on, because the consequences of not doing so will be dire. Make that commitment today.

2. MAKE YOURSELF ACCOUNTABLE

Most of us progress more readily towards our goals if there are rewards or punishments to keep us on track. Changing your eating and exercise habits have built-in rewards in terms of weight loss and improved health and well-being. However, you dramatically increase your personal accountability and thus your chances of success if you impose negative or positive consequences on your behaviors.

In my professional experience, upping the ante with a disincentive to fail is far more powerful than rewarding success. This is not an unfamiliar concept. Many of things you routinely do, such as paying taxes and showing up at work every day, are driven not by the joy of giving Uncle Sam a hunk of your paycheck or the pleasure of getting out of your warm bed at 6:00, but because of the heap of trouble you'd face if you didn't do them. Pain is a sterner taskmaster than pleasure.

The method I've had the most success with, both personally and with my patients, is to pledge a substantial amount of money to a cause you disagree with if you fail to stick with your program for a specified period of time. Don't pledge 10 bucks to the Humane Society. Pledge $250 or $1,000 to your least favorite political figure or organization. Make failing to follow through on your commitment hurt.

3. MAKE A PLAN AND WRITE IT DOWN

Once you've decided on the changes you're going to make and the consequences of blowing them, devise a plan of action. Be very specific. Get out your calendar and decide on the specific day you will start and a time period to commit to, say three weeks. Then vow to yourself *in writing* that on that date, you will, for example, cut all starches and sugars out of your diet or walk three days a week, or both. Include your incentive or disincentive (reward or punishment) in the contract, sign it, and have it witnessed by a supportive family member or friend.

In the words of the inimitable Yogi Berra, "If you don't know where you are going, you will wind up somewhere else." A written goal and a plan to achieve that goal will dramatically improve your odds of success.

4. GO PUBLIC

Blab your resolution all over the place. Tell everybody you know: spouse, kids, other family members, coworkers, friends, and enemies. This serves two purposes. First, it enlists support. Your wife will not inadvertently undermine your program by baking your favorite cookies, and your friends won't insist on taking you out to eat at the pizza joint.

Second and most important, it dramatically increases your accountability because now you're not in this alone. If you did all this in secret, nobody would be the wiser if you ate dessert. You would likely feel some internal remorse, but not enough to make you pass on the cream puffs. You might even justify to yourself that all this contract and pledge stuff is just nonsense and that you didn't really mean it. But when others are able to witness your success or failure, it's a different story. Going public is a big part of this. If you aren't willing to do it, you aren't that serious about making the changes necessary to lose weight.

5. GET READY, GET SET, GO!

Before your start date, get ready. Become very familiar with the recommended foods listed in the next chapter. Make a trip to the grocery store to purchase the poultry, fish, lean meat, eggs, vegetables, fruit, dairy products, and other things you'll be eating. I also suggest that you get rid of the items in your kitchen that are off limits, especially those that may prove to be stumbling blocks. If potato chips and jelly beans are your weakness, throw them out or donate them to a homeless shelter. (You could have one last junk food orgy, but I don't recommend it.)

Organize your exercise program. Schedule a specific time and duration to walk, do your resistance exercise routine, or whatever activity you've committed to. If your exercise plan includes working out in a gym or using specialized equipment, you obviously need to line that up beforehand.

As D day approaches, reaffirm your commitment and remind yourself that the changes you are about to make are, in the overall scheme of things, really not all that difficult—you've done much harder things in your life. You want to do this. You've promised yourself and others that you're going to do it, and as a person of character who keeps your word, you will succeed.

6. REAP THE REWARDS OF YOUR EFFORTS

Once you've honored your initial three-week commitment, evaluate your progress. Three weeks is plenty of time to break the cycle of carbohydrate cravings and overeating that your previous diet triggered. It's long enough for you to understand that this is something you can stick with, that you don't feel hungry all the time and you can still enjoy mealtimes and eating out. It's an adequate chunk of time for you to see that carving 30 minutes out of your day to exercise isn't that big a deal. Perhaps most important, you've proven to yourself that you are able to make a commitment and stick to it, and you should be very proud of yourself.

If your goal is to lose five or 10 pounds, you may have already achieved it. If you haven't hit your target weight, renew your commitment by repeating the same five steps outlined above. The only difference is that this time the process will be much easier. You know what to expect, and you know you can do it.

After you reach your goal, I urge you to continue to observe the principles of the Whitaker Wellness Weight Loss Program. Sure, you can liberalize your diet by including more low-glycemic carbohydrates. But I urge you to not make the mistake of returning to the high-starch, high-sugar diet that made you overweight in the first place. You've worked hard to get where you are, and you deserve to reap the rewards of your efforts: a lifetime of looking and feeling great.

12

WHAT SHOULD I EAT?

We've covered the fundamentals and scientific rationale of the Whitaker Wellness Weight Loss Program. Now let's get down the most important question: What should you eat? In Chapter 6, we laid the groundwork for the diet program; in the next three chapters, we'll help you put it into practice. You'll find extensive lists of foods to eat and foods to avoid. (To take the hassle out of food selection and preparation, we've created green light/red light icons for quick, at-a-glance reference.) We've also provided a three-week meal plan, complete with scores of delicious, easy-to-prepare recipes, to make this program absolutely fail-proof. Enjoy, and bon appetit!

HOW TO GUAGE PROTIONS

HERE'S A HANDY WAY TO JUDGE PORTION SIZES.

4 ounces meat = slightly larger than a deck of cards
4 ounces fish = slightly larger than a checkbook
2 tablespoons peanut butter = a Ping-Pong ball
1 ounce cheese = a pair of dice
1 ounce sliced cheese or lunchmeat = a CD
1/2 cup fruit or vegetables = a small fist
1/4 cup nuts = an adult-sized handful
1 cup chopped vegetables = a baseball
1 medium-sized piece fruit = a tennis ball

BREAKFAST

Many Americans skip breakfast thinking it will help them lose weight. Big mistake. Studies show that people who eat breakfast consume fewer calories during the day and have an easier time with weight control. The Whitaker Wellness Weight Loss Program takes this one step further. When you wake up in the morning, your body is in fat-burning mode after an overnight fast. If you avoid starches and sugars for breakfast, you can continue to burn fat throughout the morning—and the midmorning blood sugar drops that make you ravenously hungry will be history. You can accomplish this by eating 20 to 25 grams of protein and about 10 grams of carbohydrate. (If you are large-framed or physically active, you may increase your protein portion.) Here are some suggestions for your morning meal.

GREEN LIGHT—EAT
Eggs

Whole eggs, egg whites, and liquid egg-white products are protein-rich staples of the Whitaker Wellness Weight Loss Program. I recommend no more than two egg yolks per day, so use combinations of egg whites plus whole eggs. (1 egg = 2 egg whites = ¼ cup liquid egg whites). The following contain the targeted 20 to 25 grams of protein:

Whole eggs: 3–4 eggs
Egg whites: 6–8 egg whites
Liquid egg whites: ¾–1 cup
Combinations: 1 whole egg plus 4 egg whites or ½ cup egg whites
　　　　　　　 2 whole eggs plus 2 egg whites or ¼ cup egg whites

Menu Ideas

Scrambled eggs	Poached eggs
Fried eggs	Hard-boiled eggs
Soft-boiled eggs	Omelets
Frittatas	Breakfast quiche (without crust)

Half a cup of any combination of the following sautéed vegetables may be added to your egg entrées to spice them up:

Bell peppers	Spinach
Broccoli	Tomatoes
Mushrooms	Other non-starchy vegetables
Onions	

Meat and cheese may also be exchanged for one egg or two egg whites.

Turkey bacon: 3 slices	Turkey sausage: 1 ounce
Turkey ham: 1 ounce	Cheese, reduced-fat: 1 ounce

Meat, Dairy, and Vegan Options

If eggs aren't your cup of tea, try these other foods to get your 20 to 25 grams of protein for breakfast.

Reduced-fat cheese: 3 to
4 ounces
Chicken: 4 ounces
Cottage cheese,
nonfat or low-fat: ¾ cup

Tofu: 8 ounces
Turkey: 4 ounces

Fruit

Fruit is an excellent source of fiber, vitamins and other nutrients. Be aware that most fruits contain a fair amount of carbohydrates, so pay attention to portion sizes. The following portions of fruit each contain 10 or fewer grams of net carbohydrate (total carbs minus fiber).

Apple: one-half
Applesauce, unsweetened:
¼ cup
Apricots: 3
Apricots (canned, water-
packed):½ cup or 8 halves
Blueberries: ½ cup
Boysenberries: ½ cup
Cantaloupe: ½ cup
Cherries: ½ cup
Fruit cocktail (canned, water-
packed): ½ cup
Grapefruit: one-half
Grapes: ½ cup
Honeydew melon: ½ cup
Kiwifruit: 1

Mandarin oranges (canned,
water-packed): ⅓ cup
Nectarine: one-half
Orange: one-half
Peach: 1 medium
Peaches (canned, water-packed):
¾ cup
Pear: one-third
Pears (canned, water-packed): ½ cup
Pineapple: ½ cup
Plum: 1 medium
Raspberries: 1 cup
Strawberries: 1½ cups
Tangerine: 1 medium
V8 Juice (low-sodium): 8 ounces
Watermelon: ¾ cup

Meal Replacements

If you just can't stomach the thought of eating breakfast—or if you have mornings when there just isn't enough time to eat—grab a meal replacement drink or bar. Look in your health food store for a brand that contains the recommend levels of protein and carbohydrate, and make sure the ingredient list looks healthy.

Drinks

Coffee, sweetened with stevia or xylitol with a little milk or half-and-half (be wary of coffee creamers; many contain a lot of sugar)

Tea, sweetened with stevia or xylitol
Sparkling water
Water
V8 Juice, low-sodium (8 ounces, to be substituted for a serving of fruit)

RED LIGHT—DO NOT EAT

Bagels
Biscuits
Breakfast bars
Breakfast potatoes
Cold cereals
Croissants
Danishes
Doughnuts

French toast
Hash browns
Hot cereals
Jams and jellies
Juice, all types *except* low-sodium V8 Juice
Milk (a little milk in your coffee or tea is okay)

Muffins
Oatmeal
Pancakes
Pastries
Toast
Tortillas
Waffles
Yogurt, sweetened, fruit-flavored

LUNCH

Because lunches are likely to be eaten away from home, either in a restaurant or at the office, they require some advanced planning. But although the traditional sandwiches, burgers, French fries, and potato chips are off limits, you'll still have a wide array of choices that are tasty, easy to prepare (or order), and portable. Again, you'll be aiming for around 20 to 25 grams of protein and 10 grams of carbohydrates.

GREEN LIGHT—EAT
Poultry, Fish, and Other Protein Sources

The majority of the protein in your midday meal will likely come from poultry, fish, or lean meat. Eat it broiled, baked, grilled, poached, or sautéed (avoid deep fried or breaded), along with a large salad or lots of vegetables for a complete meal. The suggested serving sizes you'll need in order to get the recommended amount of protein are as follows:

Chicken: 4 ounces
Lean meat: 4 ounces
Tuna or other fish: 4 ounces

Deli meats, low-sodium: 4 ounces
Tofu: 8 ounces
Turkey: 4 ounces

Salads

Salads are a lunchtime favorite. Many of these salads are easy to make and can be found in most take-out and dine-in restaurants. Don't be tempted by the tortilla strips, croutons, crackers, and bread that commonly accompany salads—they are strictly off limits.

As far as dressings go, Italian dressing and oil and vinegar are my number one recommendations because vinegar facilitates weight loss. However, if you choose to go with another type, limit your serving to one or at most two tablespoons. Regular salad dressings are loaded with fat, and most nonfat dressings replace fat with sugars and other carbohydrates, so use in moderation. One of my favorite lunches is a piece of grilled salmon, chicken, or other protein served on top of a big green salad. Here are some protein-rich salads that are available in most restaurants (we've also included recipes for most of these and other salads):

Cobb salad	Shrimp or crab Louie
a Chef's salad	Taco salad
Chicken Caesar salad	Tuna salad
Oriental chicken salad	

Raw Vegetables

You can eat a lot of lettuce and other raw vegetables and still not exceed 10 grams of carbohydrate. Check out these amounts of uncooked vegetables that are within the 10 gram limit (of course, we aren't suggesting that eat this amount!):

Alfalfa sprouts: 12 cups	Celery: 8 stalks
Artichoke hearts: ¾ cup	Cucumbers: 1
Bell peppers: 2	Green onions: 13
Broccoli: 4 cups	Lettuce: 8+ cups
Cabbage, chopped or shredded: 2 cups	Mushrooms, sliced: 3 cups
	Snow peas: 1 cup
Carrots: 2	Spinach: 8+ cups
Cauliflower: 4 cups	Tomatoes: 2

Sandwiches

Since you won't be eating bread, you'll need to get creative if your usual noon go-to is a sandwich. Here are a few suggestions:

Bunless burgers: Top your turkey or lean beef patty with melted cheese, garnish with onions, tomato, and a pickle, and you're in business.

Tuna salad: Forget get the bread and eat tuna or chicken salad in a scooped-out tomato or avocado half.

Lettuce wraps: Wrap taco or fajita fillings in large leaves of lettuce instead of tortillas. Romaine lettuce leaves are a perfect good size, they're good for scooping, and they are more nutritious than iceberg lettuce.

Deli wraps: Use turkey, chicken, or other deli meats or your favorite reduced fat cheese slices to wrap up your sandwich fixings.

Soups

Homemade soup, made ahead in large batches and frozen in individual serving sizes, is another quick and easy lunch idea. Although recipes vary from family to family and restaurant to restaurant, here are some soups that usually come close to our nutrition guidelines. Remember to hold the crackers and bread, and if they're sparse on the meat, poultry, or seafood, order a little extra on the side.

Chili	Hot and sour soup
Chicken and vegetable soup	Minestrone (no pasta)
Clam chowder (New England or Manhattan)	Tortilla soup (pardon the oxymoron but no tortillas)
French onion soup	Vegetable beef soup (no bread)

Other Options

Healthy leftovers are always a quick and easy option, as are any of the breakfast or dinner suggestions.

Meal Replacements

If eating a good lunch isn't possible, have an appropriate meal replacement drink or bar (20 to 25 grams of protein and around 10 grams of carbs). If your meal replacement is simply a protein drink, try blending it with a little fruit for a change of pace. For amounts of fruit, see the breakfast suggestions on page 127.

Drinks

Iced tea, sweetened with stevia or xylitol	Sparkling water
	Water

RED LIGHT—DO NOT EAT

Buns	Juice	Potatoes
Bread	Pasta	Rice
Chips	Pasta salad	Sodas
Crackers	Pita	Tortillas
Desserts	Pizza	

DINNER

According to William Makepeace Thackeray, "Dinner was made for eating, not for talking." I think many of us would disagree. Dinnertime is the one opportunity we have during the day to slow down and enjoy a leisurely meal and the camaraderie of family and friends. Whether you're eating a home or dining in a restaurant, you'll have access to enjoy a wide range of healthy, tasty dinner selections. Fish, chicken, or lean meat; large servings of vegetables and salad—these foods will be so satisfying that, after a while, you won't even miss the bread, rice, and pasta.

GREEN LIGHT—EAT

Poultry, Fish, and Other Protein Sources:

Once again, your 20 to 25 grams of protein will come from the usual sources. The variety comes from the preparation: teriyaki, Thai, curry, garlic, Dijon, blackened, or any other spices to your liking. Try some of the recipes we've provided, or if you're dining out, place your order for broiled, baked, grilled, poached, or sautéed.

Chicken: 4 ounces	Fish: 4 ounces
Lean meat: 4 ounces	Shrimp: 4 ounces
Tofu: 8 ounces	Turkey: 4 ounces

Cooked Vegetables

Vegetables don't have to be boring, as you'll see from the great vegetable recipes we've included. Truth is, fresh produce, carefully selected (organic preferred) and lightly steamed or sautéed, is a delicacy in and of itself, needing only a dash of salt and pepper and perhaps a little butter or lemon juice to bring out the flavor. As you saw in the salad section above, since vegetables contain a lot of fiber, which does not raise blood sugar or provoke an insulin response, you can load your plate up with vegetables. Here are typical servings of cooked vegetables that stay within the 10-gram available carbohydrate range. (Note that dried beans are very concentrated sources of carbs.)

Broccoli: 2 cups	Corn: ⅓ cup	Spinach: 4 cups
Brussels sprouts: 11	Eggplant: 1 cup	Turnip greens: 4 cups
	Green beans: 1½ cups	Winter squash ⅔ cup
Cabbage: 2 cups	Kale: 1½ cups	Zucchini: 2 cups
Carrots: ¾ cup	Kidney beans: ¼ cup	
Chard: 3 cups	Lima beans: ⅓ cup	
Chickpeas (garbanzo beans): ¼ cup	Mushrooms: 2 cups	
	Onions: 1 cup	
	Pinto beans: ½ cup	

Drinks

Iced tea, sweetened with stevia or xylitol	Sparkling water
	Water

RED LIGHT—DO NOT EAT

Bread	Dinner rolls	Sodas
Chips	Juice	Tortillas
Couscous	Pasta	Yams
Crackers	Potatoes	
Desserts	Rice	

Snacks

Snacking is an integral part of the Whitaker Wellness Weight Loss Program. If you are hungry, a mid-morning, mid-afternoon, and even an after-dinner snack are okay. We've incorporated two snacks per day, but if you need a third one, enjoy. On the other hand, if you aren't hungry, no need to add unnecessary calories.

Unlike the main meals, your snacks should consist of about 7 grams of protein with no more than 5 grams of available carbs. Here are a few ideas to help you achieve these guidelines:

GREEN LIGHT—EAT

Celery stalks (1–2) with light cream cheese (3 tablespoons) or peanut or
almond butter (1½ tablespoons)
Edamame (boiled green soybeans), ¼ cup, dipped in soy sauce
Egg, hard-boiled or deviled, with 5 baby carrots, cherry tomatoes, or bell
pepper rings
Cottage cheese, low-fat or nonfat (¼ cup) with ¼ cup chopped peppers,
tomatoes, or peaches
Meal replacement drink: 7 grams of protein and 5 grams of carbohydrate
Nuts, raw or dry roasted: ¼ cup (peanuts, almonds, walnuts, or sunflower
seeds)
String cheese, reduced-fat (1 ounce) with 3 or 4 baby carrots, cherry
tomatoes, or bell pepper rings

RED LIGHT—DO NOT EAT

Cake	Crackers	Popcorn
Candy	Dates	Pretzels
Chips	Honey	Raisins
Chocolate	Ice cream	Rice cakes
Cookies	Juice	Sodas

Beverages

When you're thirsty during the day, drink water. Even if you're not thirsty, drink eight to ten cups of water daily—it promotes fat burning and is even more thermogenic if you drink it iced. I've explained why I'm pro-caffeine, but don't overdo it and don't mix your coffee or tea with sugar or flavored or artificial creamers that are loaded with carbohydrates. Use stevia or xylitol as a sweetener and a little milk or half-and-half, if you'd like. Green tea is an even better fat burner than coffee, plus it has a bounty of other health benefits. Regarding alcohol, one 5 ounce glass of dry wine, one ounce of hard liquor, or one light beer daily is fine. And be careful what you mix your cocktail with—tonic or soda water is fine, fruit juice and cola are not.

GREEN LIGHT—EAT

Alcohol: 1 light beer, 5-ounce glass of dry wine, or 1 ounce of spirits (drink with a meal or protein snack such as 1 ounce of cheese)
Coffee (sweetened with xylitol or stevia, with a little milk or half-and-half, if desired): within reason
Herbal teas (sweetened with xylitol or stevia): unlimited
Iced tea (sweetened with xylitol or stevia): unlimited
Sparkling water: unlimited
Tea (sweetened with xylitol or stevia: unlimited
V8 Juice (low-sodium): 8 ounces contains a meal's worth of carbohydrates
Water: unlimited

RED LIGHT—DO NOT EAT

Beer (regular)	Liquors	Sports drinks
Fruit juice	Milk	Specialty coffee drinks
Lemonade	Sodas	Wine (sweet)

RED LIGHT/GREEN LIGHT

Here's an alphabetized list of the foods you can enjoy (in the amounts indicated above) as well as the ones you need to avoid.

GREEN LIGHT—EAT

Ahi	Cabbage	Cream cheese, light
Alcohol	Canned fruit, in water	Cucumbers
Alfalfa sprouts	Cantaloupe	Deli meats
Almonds	Carrots	Edamame (soybeans)
Almond butter	Cashews	Egg whites
Apple	Cauliflower	Eggplant
Apricots	Celery	Eggs
Artichoke	Chard	Fish
Asparagus	Cheese, reduced-fat	Garlic
Avacados	Cherries	Grapefruit
Beef, lean	Chicken	Grapes
Bell peppers	Cod	Green beans
Blackberries	Coffee	Halibut
Blueberries	Cottage cheese, nonfat	Honeydew melon
Broccoli	or low-fat	Kale
Brussels sprouts	Crab	Kiwifruit

Lettuce	Peaches	Strawberries
Liquid egg white	Peanut butter	String cheese
product	Peanuts	Sunflower seeds
Low-sodium V8	Pears	Tangerines
juice	Pickles	Tea
Mandarin Oranges,	Pineapple	Tofu
water-packed	Plums	Tomatoes
Mayonnaise	Pork tenderloin	Tuna
Meal replacement	Raspberries	Turkey
drinks	Ricotta cheese,	Turkey deli slices
Milk (for coffee	part-skim	Turkey ham
only)	Salmon	Turkey sausage
Mushrooms	Salsa	Turnip greens
Mustard	Shrimp	Vinegar
Nectarines	Snow peas	Walnuts
Nuts	Soy sauce, low-sodium	Water
Olives	Spices	Watermelon
Onions	Spinach	Yogurt, plain, nonfat
Oranges	Squash	Zucchini

RED LIGHT—DO NOT EAT

Bagels	French toast	Popcorn
Biscuits	Hash browns	Potatoes
Bread	Honey	Pretzels
Breakfast bars	Hot cereals	Raisins
Breakfast	Ice cream	Rice
potatoes	Jams and jellies	Rice cakes
Cake	Juice (low-sodium V8	Sodas
Candy	acceptable)	Specialty coffee drinks
Chips	Matzo	Sports drinks
Chocolate	Milk (a little in coffee is	Sugar
Cold cereals	acceptable)	Syrup
Cookies	Muffins	Toast
Crackers	Oatmeal	Tortillas
Croissants	Pancakes	Tortilla chips
Danishes	Pasta	Waffles
Dates	Pasta salad	Yams
Dinner rolls	Pastries	Yogurt, fruit-flavored
Doughnuts	Pita bread	
English muffins	Pizza	

13

LET'S GET COOKIN'

If you like to cook—or if you've ever wanted to learn—this is the fun part. We had three goals in coming up with these recipes. First, of course, they had to fit the principles of the Whitaker Wellness Weight Loss Program. Second, they had to taste good. Last, but not least, they had to be quick and easy to prepare. We've succeeded in spades. Every meal hits the target grams of protein and carbohydrate, the dishes are simply delicious, and even beginners can handle these recipes.

Before we get to the menus and recipes, let's go over some basic information about the ingredients, cooking tools, and terms used in the recipe section, as well as a few helpful hints and how-to's.

KITCHEN EQUIPMENT

Unless your kitchen is bare-bones, you likely have most everything you'll need in the way of equipment: decent knives, a cutting board, spoons and spatulas, measuring cups and spoons, and assorted baking dishes, saucepans, and nonstick skillets. A blender or food processor comes in handy, as does a microwave, although none of these is a necessity. An outdoor grill and a George Foreman grill are also nice to have, but a broiler will do just fine. Another item that we use in a couple of recipes is a slow cooker (Crock-Pot), which is especially great for soups and one-dish meals. The best part is you can start it in the morning and come home hours later to a hot, fragrant, home-cooked dinner.

POULTRY

Skinless, boneless, individually frozen chicken breasts are a wonderful time-saver. Once you've taken out as many pieces of chicken as you need and defrosted them overnight in the refrigerator (or to speed things up, in a microwave or a bowl of cold water), they take only minutes to sauté, grill, or broil. If possible, purchase free-range chickens, which are raised in more humane conditions than "factory-farmed" poultry and are free of antibiotics and hormones. Another shortcut is to purchase whole roasted chickens, usually sold in the deli section of supermarkets. All you have to do is add a vegetable or salad, and dinner is on the table—plus the leftovers are great as snacks or in soups and other dishes.

Ground turkey, turkey deli slices, turkey "roast" (whole turkey breast), turkey sausage, turkey bacon, and turkey ham are also nice to have on hand. Don't relegate roasted turkey only to Thanksgiving. Although cooking a whole turkey takes some time, it provides a lot of meat that can be used as the basis for several meals, and you can freeze the remainder for later use. And don't forget that one of the best parts of a turkey is the rich broth you can make by boiling the bones.

FISH

We encourage you to include lots of salmon in your meals for two reasons. First, it is an exceptionally rich source of omega-3 fatty acids, and second, when you stick with wild Pacific salmon, you're able to sidestep most of the toxins that are unfortunately quite common in fish. The most worrisome of these toxins is mercury, a neurotoxin that is harmful to everyone, but especially to children. Mercury is most prevalent in large predatory species of fish such as shark, swordfish, tilefish, and king mackerel, and we recommend you avoid them altogether.

While farmed salmon isn't particularly high in mercury, it has been shown to have higher levels of other toxins such as dioxin and PCBs, plus it acquires its signature color by pigments added to its food. I'm not saying you should never eat farmed salmon, but when you have the choice, pay a little extra and go with wild salmon. Other types of seafood with low mercury levels include tilapia, herring, shrimp, pollock, cod, catfish, squid, snapper, clams, crabs, and scallops. Limit canned tuna to no more than one can a week and select light or chunk over white or albacore tuna, which, according to the FDA, contains three times more mercury.[1]

Although connoisseurs may insist on fresh fish—and we agree that it is preferable—the quality of frozen seafood can be pretty darned good. Frozen boned fish fillets and cleaned, deveined, shelled raw shrimp are great kitchen staples that, once thawed, can be prepared in a flash.

HOW-TO TIP: CLEANING AND DEVEINING SHRIMP

Hold shrimp with the tail and the outside curve facing away from you. Using sharp kitchen scissors, cut through the shell along the top of the shrimp all the way to the tail. Peel and remove the shell, keeping the tail attached and intact, if desired. Turn on kitchen faucet, hold shrimp under running water, and use a paring knife to remove the black vein. Rinse thoroughly.

BEEF AND PORK

Most of our lunches and dinners call for poultry or seafood as a protein source, but if you're a fan of beef or pork, there is no reason not to enjoy these meats. Make sure you select leaner cuts and, if you can find it, certified organic meat. The feed of these animals is free of pesticides, and, unlike much of the livestock in the U.S., they are not given hormones or antibiotics. The meat from organically raised livestock is also leaner than that of feedlot animals.

The leanest cuts of beef are tenderloin, top sirloin, top loin, round tip, and eye round. Tenderloin, boneless rib roast, and rib chops are the leanest cuts of pork and are therefore your best choices. Pork and beef sausages and hot dogs and bacon are all quite high in saturated fat and are not recommended. Lean deli ham, although a runner-up to turkey ham, is acceptable.

SOY

Tofu and soy "meats" aren't just for vegetarians. They are great sources of protein and a nice change from the usual fare. One of our particular favorites is Boca Burgers, soy hamburger patties that, although not a dead ringer for the real thing, are surprisingly close. Don't be afraid of experimenting with tofu. This protein-rich soy product tends to take on the taste of whatever it's cooked with. For stir-fries and tofu "steaks," purchase firm or extra-firm tofu. For scambled tofu, medium firmness works best.

Another type of soy we recommend that makes a good snack is edamame, boiled green soybeans that are shucked or served in the pod—just squeeze them and they pop into your mouth. A quarter cup of soybeans dipped in soy sauce makes a tasty, high-protein snack.

EGGS

Eggs and egg whites are a protein staple of the Whitaker Wellness Weight Loss Program diet. Because of their fat content, we recommend preferably one but no more than two whole eggs a day. However, you can eat all the egg whites you want, because they're almost pure protein. To save a little time, not to mention yolks, try liquid egg whites such as ReddiEgg, Quick Whites, and Egg Beaters, which are sold in the dairy or frozen foods section of your supermarket. A quarter-cup liquid egg whites equals one whole egg or two egg whites. Avoid egg substitutes.

Purchase large, cage-free, organic eggs if possible. DHA-enriched eggs are another good option—each contains 150 milligrams of omega-3 DHA fatty acids. (Gold Circle Farms is a good brand.) For do-ahead snacks, hard-boil a bunch of eggs and store them in the fridge. (See the box below.)

HOW-TO TIP: HARD-BOILING EGGS

Place desired number of raw eggs in a saucepan and fill with cold water until the water line is about an inch over the eggs. Bring the water to a boil, reduce heat to low, and simmer for 10 to 15 minutes. Remove pan from heat, pour off water, and run them under cold water to speed the cooling process. Refrigerate. The result: perfect hard-boiled eggs.

DAIRY

Low-fat or nonfat cheeses are another excellent source of protein. Reduced-fat versions of cottage, cream, ricotta, cheddar, mozzarella, Parmesan, string, and other favorites are preferable because of the rather hefty saturated fat content of cheese. Although we don't recommend milk as a beverage, a little milk or half-and-half in your coffee is just fine. When a recipe calls for butter, or you want to perk up steamed vegetables, use a little butter—it's tastier and healthier than most of the margarines out there.

We recommend that you purchase only organic dairy products. You'll be guaranteed that the milk they're made from comes from animals not treated with growth hormones and is free of pesticides and antibiotics.

VEGETABLES AND FRUIT

You are going to be eating lots of vegetables on the Whitaker Wellness Weight Loss Program, so say hello to your produce department. It's worth your while to shop around and find the store with the best fresh vegetables and fruits, and if you can locate a store that sells organic produce, so much the better. It's safer, more nutritious, and often tastier, not to mention easier on the environment.

We are big fans of the shortcuts that are popping up in the produce section. Prewashed spinach and other leafy greens with the stems removed, peeled baby carrots, broccoli and cauliflower florets, snipped herbs, and cleaned, torn lettuce are huge timesavers, and we highly recommend them. Be aware that cut produce loses nutrients more rapidly, so use it in a timely manner.

There's nothing wrong with frozen produce since it maintains most of its nutrients. Several studies show that it is as nutritious as fresh produce. Our biggest problem with it is that taste and especially texture are often inferior to fresh produce. Vegetables and fruits that lend themselves well to freezing include green peas, corn, chopped bell peppers, and leafy greens. Frozen peaches maintain decent texture, and blueberries, strawberries, and raspberries are fine if you plan to mix them with something; otherwise, they're pretty soggy. Purchase one-pound, resealable bags so you can use only what you need and keep the rest frozen for later use.

Canned vegetables we're not too crazy about—they don't hold a candle to fresh or even frozen. Exceptions, which you should keep on hand for cooking, include tomatoes, tomato paste, tomato sauce, beans, black olives, and mild green chiles. Rinse beans, olives, and chiles in a colander before using to remove excess sodium. If you like canned peaches and other fruit, purchase only water-packed and use in moderation.

HOW-TO TIP: LEMON AND LIME "ZEST"

Zesting citrus refers to removing the outermost layer of its peel. Wash fruit thoroughly, and using a fine grater or peeler, remove the skin, being careful not to take with it the white layer, or pith. (There's also a tool called a zester designed specifically for this purpose.) Once the strips are removed, finely chop and add desired amount to recipe.

OILS

Extra-virgin olive oil is the best cooking oil. In addition to being relatively stable and tolerating moderate heat, this monounsaturated oil has numerous health benefits. Its antioxidants fight free radicals, it has favorable effects on the arteries and cholesterol levels, and it may actually help relieve pain and inflammation. Olive oil makes an excellent salad dressing, and olive oil spray is good for coating skillets and baking pans.

Another healthy fat is coconut oil. Solid at room temperature, this oil can be used for baking or sautéing because it is extremely stable and will not break down under high temperatures. Unrefined organic coconut oil also contains a fatty acid called lauric acid that is being studied for its antiviral and antimicrobial effects.

Do not use the highly refined polyunsaturated vegetable oils sold in grocery stores. If you want a lighter taste than the above oils offer, look in your health food store for expeller-pressed almond, hazelnut, and other oils.

SWEETENERS

Sugars are strictly off limits in the Whitaker Wellness Weight Loss diet, and that includes not only white table sugar but also honey, brown sugar, fructose, concentrated fruit juice, and just about every other sweetener out there. In their place, we recommend stevia and xylitol. *Stevia rebaudiana* is an herb native to South America, and from it comes an intensely sweet extract sold as a dark, unrefined liquid or as a refined, concentrated liquid or powder. To sweeten your coffee or tea, the refined clear liquid extract is easiest to use. A little dab'll do ya—stevia is 200 to 250 times sweeter than sugar and too much may leave an aftertaste.

Xylitol is a sugar alcohol extracted from corn. It looks and tastes remarkably similar to white sugar, yet its effect on blood sugar is minimal. If you insist on using an artificial sweetener, the only one I'd put a tentative stamp of approval on is sucralose (Splenda). Xylitol and stevia are sold in health food stores.

NUTS AND SEEDS

Purchase nuts raw or, second best, dry roasted. One-fourth cup of almonds, peanuts, almonds, or sunflower seeds makes a great, high-protein snack. Because the oils in nuts will go rancid, keep them fresh by storing them in your freezer. In addition, make sure you purchase natural brands of almond butter and peanut butter made without hydrogenated oils.

Sprinkled on salads and other food or stirred into water, flaxseed is an excellent source of fiber, protein, and omega-3 fatty acids. Whole flaxseed can be stored indefinitely at room temperature but should be ground before eating. (A coffee grinder works great.) Once ground, flaxseed goes rancid quite quickly, so I do not recommend buying ground flaxseed. Look for flaxseed in your health food store.

14

THREE WEEKS OF MEAL PLANS AND RECIPES

Some readers will skip this chapter. They understand the principles of the program, they've grasped the dietary guidelines, and they're good to go. They know they need to avoid starches and sugars, and they've got the snacks down. They've figured out that most of their breakfast meals will consist of eggs and a little fruit, and lunches and dinners will include four ounces of fish or chicken with lots of vegetables and salad. The last thing they want is to be told exactly what to eat—they'll modify the program to suit their own tastes.

Others want to know exactly what to eat and when to eat it. It's not that they don't understand the concepts of the Whitaker Wellness Weight Loss Program—they just want to follow it to the letter. They will dog-ear the chapters on food and won't put anything in their mouth until they've checked the charts in Chapter 12. They want menus and meal plans, and they'll use them religiously.

Whether you fall into one camp or another is not a question of intelligence or perseverance; it's a matter of style. If you commit to this program, it will work for you, no matter how you choose to approach it. However, it is for the second group that we've included this chapter. Before we begin, we'd like to make a few comments on these meal plans and recipes.

PORTIONS

Throughout this book we have recommended eating 20 to 25 grams of protein and around 10 grams of available or net carbohydrates (total carbs minus fiber) at each of your three main meals. For most of you, this will be plenty of food, especially once you get into the program and are no longer under the influence of starch- and sugar-induced carbohydrate cravings. If you find this doesn't fill you up, eat more protein and lettuce, spinach, broccoli, and other low-carb vegetables. Adding extra carbs will undermine your program.

SNACKS

You'll be surprised at how satisfying these protein-dense snacks are. We've included two, one in the mid-afternoon and another after dinner, because that's all most of our patients seem to require. If you want a mid-morning snack, that is perfectly fine—have one of the suggested snacks or another of your own devising that contains around seven grams of protein and five grams of carbohydrate. On the other hand, if you don't feel hungry between meals, you are not required to eat a snack.

MEAL REPLACEMENTS

As we discussed in Chapter 12, having a supply of meal replacement drinks and bars on hand can be a huge asset to this program. When you don't have time for breakfast or lunch, all you have to do is grab a bar or stir a drink mix into water or milk (depending on carbohydrate content), and you've got a meal. Although we did not include meal replacements in the meal plan below, feel free to substitute one for any meal. A smaller serving also makes a great snack. Read labels carefully for targeted levels of protein and carbohydrate.

RECIPES

Recipes are provided for all of the items with a page reference. The nutritional analyses for each of the recipes was calculated using MasterCook software by ValuSoft, Inc.

THREE-WEEK MEAL PLAN

DAY 1

BREAKFAST
The OC Scramble (page 159)
¼ cup plain nonfat yogurt mixed with ¼ cup mandarin orange
    sections (water packed, drained) sweetened with stevia
Coffee or tea

LUNCH
Classic Chicken Caesar Salad (page 166)

MID-AFTERNOON SNACK
¼ cup raw or dry roasted almonds

DINNER
Spicy Salmon with Baby Greens (page 189)

OPTIONAL SNACK
1 stick string cheese (low-fat mozzarella)
5 baby carrots

DAY 2

BREAKFAST
Mini Breakfast Quiches (page 160)
Coffee or tea

LUNCH

Patty Melt with Caramelized Onions (page 167)

Large tossed salad (2 cups lettuce with ½ cup cucumbers, tomatoes, and/or green peppers or other vegetables and 1 tablespoon salad dressing)

MID-AFTERNOON SNACK

Heavenly Deviled Egg (page 187)

½ cup cherry tomatoes

DINNER

"Spaghetti" and Italian Sausage (page 190)

Small side salad (1 cup lettuce)

OPTIONAL SNACK

2 celery stalks with 1½ tablespoons peanut butter

DAY 3

BREAKFAST

Bacon 'n eggs (3 slices turkey bacon and 2 fried, scrambled, soft-boiled, or poached eggs)

½ grapefruit

Coffee or tea

LUNCH

Sopa de Pollo (page 168)

Tossed salad (2 cups lettuce with 1 tablespoon dressing)

MID-AFTERNOON SNACK

2 stalks celery with 3 tablespoons light cream cheese

DINNER

Halibut Dijon (page 192)

Zucchini-Parmesan Sauté (page 214)

OPTIONAL SNACK
Raspberry-Lemon Delight (page 188)

DAY 4

BREAKFAST
¾ cup low-fat or nonfat cottage cheese
½ cup blueberries
Coffee or tea

LUNCH
Crunchy Tuna Salad (page 169)
1 sliced tomato

MID-AFTERNOON SNACK
¼ cup sunflower seeds

DINNER
Southwestern Chicken Fajitas (page 194)
Gringo Guacamole (page 195)

OPTIONAL SNACK
Hard-boiled egg
½ red bell pepper, sliced

DAY 5

BREAKFAST
Ham & Cheese Omelet (page 161)
6 ounces low-sodium V8 Juice
Coffee or tea

LUNCH
Chopped Chinese Chicken Salad (page 170)

MID-AFTERNOON SNACK
Spicy cottage cheese (¼ cup low-fat or nonfat cottage cheese with
¼ cup salsa)

DINNER
Shrimp Shish Kabobs (page 193)
Green Beans Extraordinaire (page 196)
Tossed salad (2 cups lettuce or spinach with 1 tablespoon dressing)

OPTIONAL SNACK
2 celery stalks with 1½ tablespoons peanut butter

DAY 6

BREAKFAST
Tex-Mex Eggs (page 162)
Coffee or tea

LUNCH
California Chili (page 171)
½ cup cucumber slices

MID-AFTERNOON SNACK
¼ cup edamame (soybeans) dipped in soy sauce

DINNER
Easy Baked Salmon (page 197)
Steamed Broccoli with Lemon Sauce (page 198)

OPTIONAL SNACK
¼ cup walnuts

DAY 7

BREAKFAST
2 ounces smoked salmon, 1 hard-boiled egg, 1 ounce reduced-fat
cheese
½ orange
Coffee or tea

LUNCH
Oriental Beef Salad (page 172)

MID-AFTERNOON SNACK
¼ cup dry roasted peanuts

DINNER
Bayside Broiled Chicken (page 199)
Lemon Pepper Asparagus (page 200)
Green salad

OPTIONAL SNACK
¼ cup nonfat or low-fat cottage cheese with ¼ cup peaches (packed in
water or light syrup)

DAY 8

BREAKFAST
Omelet Florentine (page 163)
⅓ cup plain nonfat yogurt with ⅓ cup raspberries, sweetened with
stevia
Coffee or tea

LUNCH
Connie's Quick & Easy Stew (page 173)
½ avocado

MID-AFTERNOON SNACK
2 stalks of celery with 3 tablespoons light cream cheese

DINNER
Seared Ahi Salad with Wasabi Dressing (page 201)
¼ cup mandarin orange sections (in water or light syrup)

OPTIONAL SNACK
¼ cup sunflower seeds

DAY 9

BREAKFAST
Scrambled eggs and cheese (1 whole egg plus 4 egg whites or ½ cup
    liquid egg whites and 1 ounce grated reduced-fat cheese)
⅔ cup raspberries
Coffee or tea

LUNCH
Just Beachy Fish Tacos (page 174)

MID-AFTERNOON SNACK
¼ cup walnuts

DINNER
Joe's Special (page 204)
Sliced tomatoes (½ tomato per person)

OPTIONAL SNACK
Raspberry-Lemon Delight (page 188)

DAY 10

BREAKFAST
Turkey rolls (3 ounces turkey deli slices rolled around 1 ounce string
    cheese)

1 apricot
Coffee or tea

LUNCH
Mushroom Burger (page 175)
Spinach and tomato salad (2 cups spinach plus half a tomato and
1 teaspoon salad dressing)

MID-AFTERNOON SNACK
Hard-boiled egg
½ cup cherry tomatoes

DINNER
Salmon Patties on Field Greens (page 202)

OPTIONAL SNACK
Crunchy cottage cheese (¼ cup low-fat or nonfat cottage cheese
with ½ cup chopped red bell pepper)

DAY 11

BREAKFAST
Green Eggs and Ham (page 164)
6 ounces low-sodium V8 Juice
Coffee or tea

LUNCH
Classic Cobb Salad (page 176)

MID-AFTERNOON SNACK
¼ cup almonds

DINNER
Bayou Shrimp (page 205)
Tossed green salad (2 cups lettuce, ¼ tomato with 1 teaspoon
dressing)

OPTIONAL SNACK
¼ cup nonfat cottage cheese
½ cup strawberries

DAY 12

BREAKFAST
2 ounces smoked salmon, 1 hard-boiled egg, and 1 ounce reduced-fat
   cheese
½ cup honeydew melon balls
Coffee or tea

LUNCH
Tuna Stuffed Tomatoes (page 177)

MID-AFTERNOON SNACK
1 stick string cheese (low-fat mozzarella)
5 baby carrots

DINNER
Grilled chicken breast (marinated in Italian dressing)
Sautéed zucchini
Broccoli-Olive Salad (page 206)

OPTIONAL SNACK
¼ cup sunflower seeds

DAY 13

BREAKFAST
¾ cup low-fat or nonfat cottage cheese
½ cup raspberries
Coffee or tea

LUNCH
Chicken or turkey sausage (4 ounces) with mustard and sauerkraut
Cool and Crunchy Coleslaw (page 178)

MID-AFTERNOON SNACK
Hard-boiled egg
½ cup bell pepper rings

DINNER
Pacific Pork Carnitas (page 207)
Tossed green salad (2 cups lettuce, ¼ tomato with 1 teaspoon dressing)

OPTIONAL SNACK
Raspberry-Lemon Delight (page 188)

DAY 14

BREAKFAST
Scrambled ham and eggs (1 whole egg plus 4 egg whites or ½ cup
    Egg Beaters and 1 ounce turkey ham)
1 tangerine
Coffee or tea

LUNCH
Seafood Lettuce Wraps (page 179)
1 pear

MID-AFTERNOON SNACK
¼ cup dry roasted peanuts

DINNER
Cashew Chicken (page 215)
Raw snow peas (½ cup)

OPTIONAL SNACK
Spicy cottage cheese (¼ cup low-fat or nonfat cottage cheese with
    ¼ cup salsa)

DAY 15

BREAKFAST
Beachcomber Tofu Scramble (page 165)
1 small wedge cantaloupe

LUNCH
Black and White Chili (page 180)

MID-AFTERNOON SNACK
2 celery stalks with 1½ tablespoons peanut butter

DINNER
Poached Salmon with Cucumber Sauce (page 216)
Wilted Greens (page 208)

OPTIONAL SNACK
1 stick string cheese (low-fat mozzarella)
5 baby carrots

DAY 16

BREAKFAST
Turkey rolls (3 ounces turkey deli slices rolled around 1 ounce string cheese)
½ cup strawberries
Coffee or tea

LUNCH
Greek Shrimp Salad (page 181)

MID-AFTERNOON SNACK
Crunchy cottage cheese (¼ cup low-fat or nonfat cottage cheese with ½ cup diced red bell pepper)

DINNER
Teriyaki Chicken with Mushroom Gravy (page 209)
Whitaker Wellness Mashed "Potatoes" (page 217)

OPTIONAL SNACK
¼ cup walnuts

DAY 17

BREAKFAST
The OC Scramble (page 159)
¼ cup plain nonfat yogurt mixed with ¼ cup raspberries sweetened
    with stevia
Coffee or tea

LUNCH
Chef Priscilla's Chicken Satay with Peanut Sauce (page 182)

MID-AFTERNOON SNACK
Heavenly Deviled Eggs (page 187)
½ cup cherry tomatoes

DINNER
Lettuce Wrapped Tacos (page 218)

OPTIONAL SNACK
1 celery stalk with 1½ tablespoons almond butter

DAY 18

BREAKFAST
Scrambled eggs and cheese (1 whole egg plus 4 egg whites or ½ cup
    Egg Beaters and 1 ounce grated reduced-fat cheese)
½ cup blackberries
Coffee or tea

LUNCH

Almost all-American burger (4 ounce turkey or lean beef burger, no bun, with lettuce leaf, onion and tomato slice, and 1 teaspoon each mayonnaise, mustard, and ketchup)

3 celery stalks and 3 bell pepper rings with 1 tablespoon ranch dressing for dipping

MID-AFTERNOON SNACK

¼ cup dry roasted peanuts

DINNER

Sole a l'Orange (page 210)

Brussels sprouts (1 cup)

OPTIONAL SNACK

Raspberry-Lemon Delight (page 188)

DAY 19

BREAKFAST

¾ cup low-fat or nonfat cottage cheese

½ cup raspberries

Coffee or tea

LUNCH

Hot and Sour Soup (page 184)

MID-AFTERNOON SNACK

2 celery stalks with 1½ tablespoons peanut butter

DINNER

Spinach-Cheese Stuffed Chicken Breasts (page 211)

Tossed salad (2 cups lettuce, ¼ cup tomato with 1 teaspoon dressing)

OPTIONAL SNACK

¼ cup nonfat cottage cheese

½ cup raspberries

DAY 20

BREAKFAST

Scrambled egg whites (7 egg whites scrambled with ¼ cup each
onion and green pepper)

1 apricot

Coffee or tea

LUNCH

Signature Chef's Salad (page 186)

MID-AFTERNOON SNACK

¼ cup almonds

DINNER

Shrimp and Broccoli Stir-Fry (page 212)

Spinach Salad (2 cups) with dressing

OPTIONAL SNACK

Spicy cottage cheese (¼ cup low-fat or nonfat cottage cheese with
¼ cup salsa)

DAY 21

BREAKFAST

Turkey rolls (3 ounces turkey deli slices rolled around 1 ounce string
cheese)

½ cup strawberries

Coffee or tea

LUNCH

Salmon-Avocado Salad (page 185)

MID-AFTERNOON SNACK

2 celery stalks with 3 tablespoons light cream cheese

DINNER

Roasted Chicken (page 213)
Garlicky Greens (page 191)
Large tossed salad

OPTIONAL SNACK

¼ cup dry-roasted peanuts

RECIPES

The OC Scramble
An easy way to start your day

Yield: 2 servings
Start to finish: 10 minutes

1	teaspoon extra virgin olive oil
½	cup mushrooms, chopped
½	cup red or green bell pepper, diced
12	egg whites or 1½ cups liquid egg whites
1	tablespoon water
1	tablespoon Parmesan cheese, grated
¼	teaspoon ground pepper
	Dash salt

Heat olive oil in a medium nonstick skillet over medium-high heat. Add the peppers and mushrooms to skillet and sauté, stirring often, for 2 to 3 minutes, until tender. Mix the egg whites, water, cheese, pepper, and salt in a small bowl, and pour into skillet. Cook for another 1 to 2 minutes, stirring until eggs are set.

Per serving: calories 147, protein 23 g, carbohydrates 6 g, fiber 1 g, fat 3 g (monounsaturated 2 g, polyunsaturated trace, saturated 1 g), sodium 510 mg

BREAKFAST

Mini Breakfast Quiches
A tasty breakfast that's good on the go

Yield: 2 servings
Start to finish: 30 minutes

½	cup tomato, seeded and finely chopped
6	egg whites or ¾ cup liquid egg whites
½	cup reduced-fat cheddar cheese, shredded
½	cup onion, finely chopped
¼	teaspoon ground pepper
	Olive oil spray

Preheat the oven to 350 degrees. Drain the tomato on paper towels to remove as much water as possible. In a bowl mix together the egg whites, cheese, onion, tomato, and pepper. Line a 6-cup muffin tin with foil cups and spray lightly with olive oil. Spoon the egg mixture evenly into the foil cups. Bake for 20 minutes, or until a toothpick or knife placed in the center of the quiche comes out clean.

NOTE: Try this versatile recipe with mushrooms, bell peppers, mild green chiles, spinach, broccoli, or other vegetables in place of the tomatoes and onions. Mini Breakfast Quiches may be made ahead and reheated.

Per serving: calories 141, protein 22 g, carbohydrates 8 g, fiber 1 g, fat 2 g (monounsaturated 1 g, polyunsaturated trace, saturated 1 g), sodium 397 mg

Ham & Cheese Omelet
Back to basics

Yield: 1 serving
Start to finish: 10 minutes

4	egg whites or ½ cup Egg Beaters or other egg white product
	Dash ground black pepper
1	teaspoon water
½	teaspoon butter
¼	cup diced turkey ham
1	tablespoon shredded reduced-fat cheddar cheese

In a small bowl beat the eggs with the pepper and water with a fork until well blended. Heat an 8-inch nonstick skillet over medium-high heat. Add the butter and swirl around until pan is coated. Pour in the eggs and tip the skillet to distribute the eggs evenly over the bottom of the pan. As the eggs begin to set, tilt the pan and lift the edge of the omelet with a fork, allowing the uncooked eggs to slide underneath. When the omelet is set, sprinkle ham and cheese on top and let it stand over the heat for several seconds to melt the cheese, warm the ham, and brown the bottom. Slide onto a plate, fold, and serve.

Per serving: calories 164, protein 26 g, carbohydrates 2 g, fiber trace, fat 5 g (monounsaturated 1 g, polyunsaturated 1 g, saturated 1 g), sodium 842 mg

BREAKFAST

Tex-Mex Eggs
A spicy twist on a morning favorite

Yield: 4 servings
Start to finish: 20 minutes

4	eggs
8	egg whites or 1 cup liquid egg whites
	Dash salt
¼	teaspoon ground pepper
1	teaspoon extra virgin olive oil
1	onion, chopped
1	green bell pepper, chopped
1	cup shredded reduced-fat cheddar cheese
1	cup salsa

Combine the eggs, egg whites, salt, and pepper in a small bowl and mix well. In a large nonstick skillet, heat the olive oil over medium heat. Add the onion and green bell pepper and sauté, stirring frequently, for 3 to 4 minutes until crisp-tender. Pour in the egg mixture and cook, stirring occasionally, until the eggs are just set, about 3 minutes. Stir in the cheese. Serve with salsa.

Per serving: calories 195, protein 21 g, carbohydrates 10 g, fiber 2 g, fat 8 g (monounsaturated 3 g, polyunsaturated 3 g, saturated 3 g), sodium 687 mg

Omelet Florentine

Full of spinach, cheese, and great taste

Yield: 1 serving
Start to finish: 15 minutes

3	egg whites or ⅓ cup liquid egg whites
1	egg
	Dash pepper
1	teaspoon water
	Olive oil spray
1	cup fresh spinach
½	teaspoon butter
2	tablespoons shredded reduced-fat cheddar cheese

Beat the egg whites, egg, pepper, and water together with a fork until well mixed. Heat an 8-inch nonstick skillet over medium-high heat. Spray with olive oil and add the spinach, stirring until the spinach wilts, about 2 minutes. Remove the spinach and dab it with a paper towel to remove excess water. Add the butter to the skillet and swirl around until well coated. Pour the eggs in and tip the skillet to distribute the eggs evenly over the bottom of the pan. As the eggs begin to set, tilt the pan and lift the edge of the omelet with a fork, allowing the uncooked eggs to slide underneath. When the omelet is set, sprinkle the cheese on top and add the spinach. Warm until cheese is melted and omelet is browned. Slide onto a plate, fold, and serve.

Per serving: calories 164, protein 20 g, carbohydrates 3 g, fiber 1 g, fat 7 g (monounsaturated 3 g, polyunsaturated 1 g, saturated 3 g), sodium 349 mg

BREAKFAST

Green Eggs and Ham

Inspired by Dr. Seuss

Yield: 1 serving
Start to finish: 15 minutes

¾	cup finely chopped broccoli
3	teaspoons water
1	egg
2	egg whites or ¼ cup liquid egg whites
	Dash black pepper
½	teaspoon butter
2	ounces turkey ham, chopped

Heat an 8-inch nonstick skillet over medium heat. Add the broccoli and 2 teaspoons of water, cover, and cook for 1 or 2 minutes, or until the broccoli is bright green and crisp-tender. Remove from the pan and drain. Beat the egg, egg whites, 1 teaspoon water, and black pepper in a small bowl. Melt the butter in the skillet over medium heat. Return the broccoli to pan along with the ham, spreading them out evenly. Immediately pour the egg mixture over the broccoli. Tilt the pan and lift the edges of the eggs to allow uncooked eggs to run underneath. Cook for several minutes until the eggs are set and browned. Slide or remove from pan with a spatula, fold, and serve.

Per serving: calories 195, protein 25 g, carbohydrates 5 g, fiber 2 g, fat 8 g (monounsaturated 2 g, polyunsaturated 3 g, saturated 3 g), sodium 753 mg

Beachcomber Tofu Scramble
A nice change from eggs for breakfast

Yield: 2 servings

Start to finish: 15 minutes

1	teaspoon extra virgin olive oil
12	ounces medium-firm tofu, cut into ½-inch cubes
1	clove garlic, peeled and minced
½	onion, chopped
½	red or green bell pepper, chopped
½	cup chopped spinach
	Dash salt
	Dash pepper
2	ounces reduced-fat cheese, grated

In a large nonstick skillet, heat the olive oil over medium-high heat. Add the tofu and cook for 5 minutes, stirring often. Add the garlic, onion, bell pepper, and spinach and cook, stirring frequently, for another 3 to 5 minutes, or until the tofu is hot and the spinach is wilted. Season with the salt and pepper. Add the cheese and stir until melted.

Per serving: calories 223, protein 21 g, carbohydrates 11 g, fiber 2 g, fat 12 g (monounsaturated 4 g, polyunsaturated 5 g, saturated 3 g), sodium 328 mg

Classic Chicken Caesar Salad

An old favorite packed with protein

Yield: 4 servings

Start to finish: 20 minutes

1	clove garlic, peeled and minced
2	tablespoons lemon juice
1½	teaspoons Dijon mustard
1½	teaspoons Worcestershire sauce
½	teaspoon anchovy paste, optional
½	teaspoon salt
¼	teaspoon ground black pepper
3	tablespoons extra virgin olive oil
16	cups chopped lettuce
2	cups diced cooked chicken
¼	cup grated Parmesan cheese

In a large mixing bowl, add garlic, lemon juice, mustard, Worcestershire sauce, anchovy paste, salt, and pepper, and blend well. Slowly pour in the olive oil and stir with a whisk until mixture thickens. Add lettuce, chicken, and cheese to bowl and toss with dressing.

Per serving: calories 282, protein 27 g, carbohydrates 10 g, fiber 4 g, fat 16 g (monounsaturated 9 g, polyunsaturated 2 g, saturated 3 g), sodium 476 mg

Patty Melt with Caramelized Onions
Cheeseburger, please—hold the bun

Yield: 2 servings
Start to finish: 15 minutes

1	teaspoon extra virgin olive oil
½	large onion, sliced
2	(4-ounce) ground turkey burgers
2	ounces reduced-fat cheddar cheese, thinly sliced

In a large, nonstick skillet, heat the olive oil over medium heat. Add the onions and cook for about 5 minutes, stirring often, or until tender and golden brown. Keep warm.

Cook the turkey burgers over medium heat until cooked through. Preheat the broiler. Divide grilled onions evenly on burgers. Top with cheese. Place on a cookie sheet and cook under broiler until cheese melts, 1 to 2 minutes.

NOTE: For a quick vegetarian option, substitute one and a half frozen Boca Burgers or another soy protein patty for turkey burger. Prepare per package instructions.

Per serving: calories 248, protein 27 g, carbohydrates 3 g, fiber trace g, fat 14 g (monounsaturated 6 g, polyunsaturated 3 g, saturated 4 g), sodium 281 mg

Sopa de Pollo
Tortilla soup without the tortillas

Yield: 8 servings
Start to finish: 45 minutes

5	cups low-sodium chicken broth
2	cups water
1	(14½ ounces) can low-sodium tomatoes, chopped, with juice
1	medium onion, chopped
3	cloves garlic, peeled and minced
⅓	cup chopped cilantro
1	to 2 chipotle chilies canned in adobo sauce, chopped, with a little sauce (use with care—chipotles are hot!)
3	cups cooked chicken, diced
¾	cup grated reduced-fat cheddar or Monterey Jack cheese
1	avocado, chopped
2	limes, quartered

In a large saucepan, place broth, water, tomatoes (and their juice), onion, garlic, cilantro, chilies, and chicken. Bring to a boil, reduce heat, and simmer for 30 minutes. Garnish with cheese and avocado. Serve with lime wedges.

Per serving: calories 206, protein 28 g, carbohydrates 9 g, fiber 2 g, fat 7 g (monounsaturated 3 g, polyunsaturated 1 g, saturated 2 g), sodium 463 mg

Crunchy Tuna Salad

A tasty variation on a timeless classic

Yield: 2 servings

Start to finish: 10 minutes

1	(6-ounce) can chunk light tuna in water, drained
½	cup chopped celery
¼	cup light mayonnaise
2	tablespoons chopped onion
⅛	teaspoon seasoned salt
⅛	teaspoon ground black pepper
¼	cup chopped almonds
2	romaine lettuce leaves

Combine the tuna, celery, mayonnaise, onion, salt, and pepper in a medium bowl and mix well. Just before serving, stir in the almonds. Serve on lettuce leaves.

Per serving: calories 283, protein 26 g, carbohydrates 11 g, fiber 3 g, fat 16 g (monounsaturated 8 g, polyunsaturated 5 g, saturated 2 g), sodium 551 mg

LUNCH

Chopped Chinese Chicken Salad
Asian-American fusion at its finest

Yield: 4 servings
Start to finish: 20 minutes

2	tablespoons extra virgin olive oil
1	tablespoon sesame oil
1	tablespoon low-sodium soy sauce
3	tablespoons lemon juice
2	cloves garlic, peeled and minced
1	teaspoon grated lemon peel
¾	pound cooked chicken breast, coarsely chopped
5	cups coarsely chopped spinach
5	cups coarsely chopped romaine lettuce
4	green onions, chopped
1	cup fresh bean sprouts
2	tablespoons toasted sesame seeds

Combine the oils, soy sauce, lemon juice, garlic, and lemon peel in medium bowl and mix well. Add the chicken and let sit in refrigerator for 10 minutes.

Mix the spinach, romaine, green onions, and bean sprouts in a large serving bowl. Just before serving, add the chicken mixture and toss with sesame seeds.

Per serving: calories 258, protein 23 g, carbohydrates 9 g, fiber 4 g, fat 15 g (monounsaturated 7 g, polyunsaturated 5 g, saturated 2 g), sodium 236 mg

California Chili
Chipotle chilies give this standard a smoky kick

Yield: 4 servings
Start to finish: 1 hour, 30 minutes (minimum)

1	teaspoon extra virgin olive oil
1	pound ground turkey
¾	cup chopped onion
¾	cup chopped green bell pepper
1	clove garlic, peeled and minced
½	cup sliced ripe olives
1	(14½-ounce) can low-sodium tomatoes, chopped, with juice
¼	cup tomato paste
3	cups water
2	tablespoons chili powder
½	teaspoon cumin
1	to 2 chipotle chiles canned in adobo sauce (to taste—they're very hot) or ¼ to ½ teaspoon red pepper flakes
4	tablespoons chopped cilantro
4	tablespoons shredded reduced-fat cheddar cheese

In a large stockpot or Dutch oven, heat the olive oil over medium-high heat. Add the ground turkey, onion, and bell pepper and cook until browned. Drain. Add the garlic, olives, tomatoes, tomato paste, water, chili powder, cumin, chiles, and cilantro. Stir well and bring to a boil. Reduce the heat to low and simmer for at least 1 hour. (Chili can be cooked up to 4 hours for added flavor. Add water as needed.) Serve sprinkled with cheese.

NOTE: This is a great recipe for slow cooker cooking. After browning the turkey, onion, and bell pepper in the nonstick skillet, transfer the remaining ingredients with the exception of the cheese to a slow cooker. Cook on low 10 to 12 hours or on high for 5 to 6 hours.

Per serving: calories 298, protein 25 g, carbohydrates 16 g, fiber 5 g, fat 16 g (monounsaturated 7 g, polyunsaturated 3 g, saturated 5 g), sodium 487 mg

Oriental Beef Salad

Here's a salad even meat lovers will enjoy

Yield: 4 servings

Start to finish: 45 minutes (in addition to overnight marinating after broiling)

LUNCH

1	pound sirloin steak, trimmed of fat
1	tablespoon low-sodium soy sauce
½	teaspoon ground black pepper
2	green onions, sliced
	Zest of 1 lime (grated peel)
3	tablespoons lime juice
½	teaspoon xylitol
¼	teaspoon red pepper flakes
12	cups mixed field greens
1	cucumber, peeled and thinly sliced
2	tablespoons fresh mint, chopped
1	tablespoons sesame oil
1	tablespoon extra virgin olive oil

Preheat the broiler and position the rack in the upper third of the oven. Rub the steak with soy sauce and black pepper and place on a broiler pan. Broil for 14 to 16 minutes, turning once. Remove from the oven and cool for 5 minutes.

While the meat is cooling, combine the green onions, lime zest, lime juice, xylitol, and red pepper flakes in a shallow dish or pan. Slice the steak into thin, bite-sized pieces and add to the marinade in the shallow dish. Add any accumulated juices, toss well, making sure to thoroughly coat each piece. Cover and refrigerate overnight.

When ready to serve, place field greens, cucumber slices, and mint in a salad bowl. Add the steak. Combine the remaining marinade with the oils and drizzle over the salad. Toss gently and serve immediately.

Per serving: calories 341, protein 24 g, carbohydrates 11 g, fiber 4 g, fat 23 g (monounsaturated 10 g, polyunsaturated 3 g, saturated 7 g), sodium 227 mg

Connie's Quick & Easy Stew

From the Whitaker's kitchen straight to yours

Yield: 6 servings
Start to finish: 1 hour, 30 minutes

1	teaspoon extra virgin olive oil
1	pound extra lean ground turkey
2	cloves garlic, peeled and minced
1	large onion, chopped
2	medium carrots, sliced ½-inch thick
3	stalks celery, sliced ½-inch thick
6	cups low-sodium beef broth
1	(14½-ounce) can low-sodium tomatoes, chopped, with juice
2	teaspoons Worcestershire sauce
2	bay leaves
⅛	teaspoon red pepper flakes
½	teaspoon ground black pepper
¼	teaspoon dried oregano

Heat the olive oil in a large, heavy saucepan or Dutch oven over medium heat. Add the ground turkey and sauté, stirring frequently, until cooked through, about 10 minutes. Drain and return to saucepan. Add the garlic, onion, carrots, and celery to the pan and cook for another 5 minutes, stirring occasionally. Pour the beef broth into the saucepan and add the tomatoes, Worcestershire sauce, bay leaves, red pepper flakes, black pepper, and oregano. Cook for 45 minutes to 1 hour, stirring occasionally and adding water to achieve desired consistency. Stew should be thick and hearty.

NOTE: This may also be prepared in a slow cooker. After browning the turkey, place all ingredients in slow cooker and cook on low for 8 to 10 hours.

Per serving: calories 202, protein 28 g, carbohydrates 10 g, fiber 2 g, fat 8 g (monounsaturated 4 g, polyunsaturated 2 g, saturated 2 g), sodium 144 mg

Just Beachy Fish Tacos
A light, healthy version of a Newport Beach favorite

Yield: 4 servings

Start to finish: 20 minutes

2	tablespoons lime juice
½	teaspoon chili powder
½	teaspoon salt
4	(4-ounce) cod fillets, or other white fish
8	whole romaine lettuce leaves
1	large avocado, thinly sliced
1	cup chopped tomatoes
2	green onions, thinly sliced
1	cup salsa
8	tablespoons grated reduced-fat cheddar cheese
1	lime, cut into 4 wedges

Mix the lime juice, chili powder, and salt together in a bowl and pour over the fish. Cover and refrigerate for 10 minutes while preparing the vegetables.

Preheat the broiler with the rack set 3 to 4 inches from the heat. Broil the fish for 4 to 6 minutes. (If the fillets are thin, you won't need to turn them. If they're thick, turn after 3 minutes.) Break the fish into chunks. Using lettuce leaves like tortillas, place fish fillets in lettuce leaves and top with avocado, tomatoes, onions, salsa, and cheese. Squeeze lime juice over tacos for flavor.

Per serving: calories 239, protein 26 g, carbohydrates 14 g, fiber 4 g, fat 10 g (monounsaturated 5 g, polyunsaturated 1 g, saturated 2 g), sodium 444 mg

Mushroom Burger

An easy way to jazz up a bunless burger

Yield: 4 servings
Start to finish: 20 minutes

3	tablespoons low-sodium soy sauce (divided use)
1	clove garlic, minced
1	pound lean ground turkey (or beef)
1	teaspoon extra virgin olive oil
6	cups sliced mushrooms

Mix 2 tablespoons of the soy sauce and the garlic into the ground turkey and shape into 4 patties about ¾-inch thick. Heat a large nonstick skillet over medium-high heat. Add the patties and sauté for 5 to 7 minutes per side. When done, remove from pan, pour off the juices, and keep warm.

Add olive oil to pan, then sauté the mushrooms, stirring often, for 3 to 4 minutes. Add the remaining tablespoon soy sauce to the mushrooms and continue cooking until crisp-tender. To serve, place the patties on a plate and spoon the mushrooms over top.

Per serving: calories 214, protein 23 g, carbohydrates 6 g, fiber 1 g, fat 11 g (monounsaturated 4 g, polyunsaturated 3 g, saturated 3 g), sodium 561 mg

Classic Cobb Salad

An oldie but goodie

Yield: 4 servings
Start to finish: 15 minutes

12	cups shredded romaine lettuce
2	medium tomatoes, diced
1	large avocado, diced
4	slices turkey bacon, cooked and chopped
3	tablespoons crumbled blue cheese
1	cup chilled and diced cooked chicken breast
2	hard-boiled eggs, chopped
4	tablespoons blue cheese salad dressing

Divide the lettuce evenly in four individual serving bowls and arrange the remaining ingredients in order in rows on top. Serve with 1 tablespoon blue cheese dressing per salad.

Per serving: calories 381, protein 26 g, carbohydrates 12 g, fiber 5 g, fat 27 g (monounsaturated 11 g, polyunsaturated 7 g, saturated 6 g), sodium 515 mg

Tuna Stuffed Tomatoes

Tasty tuna in a tomato shell

Yield: 2 servings
Start to finish: 10 minutes

2	whole tomatoes, red ripe, beefsteak-type
1	(6-ounce) can chunk light tuna in water, drained
2	tablespoons mayonnaise
2	green onions, chopped
⅓	cup chopped dill pickle
¼	cup sliced black olives

Cut the tops off the tomatoes and scoop out the insides with a spoon. Place the tuna in a bowl and add the mayonnaise, green onions, pickle, and olives and gently stir until well mixed. Spoon the tuna mixture into the tomato shells and serve.

Per serving: calories 242, protein 21 g, carbohydrates 9 g, fiber 3 g, fat 15 g (monounsaturated 5 g, polyunsaturated 6 g, saturated 2 g), sodium 828 mg

LUNCH

Cool and Crunchy Coleslaw
A simple, make-ahead slaw

Yield: 4 servings
Start to finish: 45 minutes

½	cup plain nonfat yogurt
¼	cup low-fat mayonnaise
½	teaspoon dry mustard
½	teaspoon seasoned salt
⅛	teaspoon ground black pepper
1	pound green cabbage (about 12 cups), finely shredded or chopped
¼	cup chopped green onion

Mix the yogurt, mayonnaise, mustard, seasoned salt, and pepper in a large bowl. Toss with the cabbage and onion. Chill for 30 minutes before serving.

Per serving: calories 68, protein 2 g, carbohydrates 10 g, fiber 3 g, fat 3 g (monounsaturated 1 g, polyunsaturated 2 g, saturated 1 g), sodium 266 mg

Seafood Lettuce Wraps
A little taste of the ocean

Yield: 4 servings
Start to finish: 15 minutes

6	ounces tiny boiled canned shrimp, rinsed, drained, chopped
9	ounces crabmeat, fresh or canned, or imitation crab (surimi), shredded
1	cup chopped celery
⅓	cup chopped green onion
½	cup light mayonnaise
3	tablespoons chopped parsley
1	teaspoon Mrs. Dash salt-free seasoning (or more to taste)
¼	teaspoon onion powder
¼	teaspoon garlic powder
⅛	teaspoon ground black pepper
8	romaine lettuce leaves

In a medium bowl, combine the shrimp, crab, celery, onion, mayonnaise, parsley, Mrs. Dash seasoning, onion powder, garlic powder, and black pepper and stir until well blended. Place 2 lettuce leaves on each plate. Spoon the seafood mixture onto lettuce and eat taco-style.

Per serving: calories 187, protein 20 g, carbohydrates 7 g, fiber 1 g, fat 7 g (monounsaturated 2 g, polyunsaturated 4 g, saturated 1 g), sodium 487 mg

Black and White Chili

Decidedly different—but delicious

Yield: 4 servings

Start to finish: 45 minutes

1	teaspoon extra virgin olive oil
¾	pound chicken breast without skin (or turkey breast), cut into ½-inch cubes
1	medium onion, chopped
1	clove garlic, peeled and finely chopped
1	(3½-ounce) can green chile peppers, chopped
3	cups low-sodium chicken broth
1	tablespoon chili powder
1	cup cooked black beans, rinsed and drained

Heat the oil in a medium saucepan over medium-high heat. Cook the chicken or turkey, onion, and garlic, stirring occasionally, until the meat is cooked through and the onion is tender. Stir in the chile peppers, chicken broth, chili powder, and black beans. Heat to boiling; reduce the heat to low. Cover and simmer for 30 minutes, stirring occasionally.

Per serving: calories 237, protein 25 g, carbohydrates 16 g, fiber 5 g, fat 7 g (monounsaturated 3 g, polyunsaturated 2 g, saturated 2 g), sodium 658 mg

Greek Shrimp Salad

Not your run-of-the-mill Greek salad

Yield: 4 servings

Start to finish: 20 minutes

2	tablespoons balsamic vinegar
2	tablespoons extra virgin olive oil
1	clove garlic, peeled and minced
¼	teaspoon ground black pepper
¼	teaspoon seasoned salt, or salt substitute
12	cups chopped lettuce
2	tomatoes, sliced
1	cucumber, sliced
½	cup thinly sliced red onion
1	cup black olives, pitted (kalamata preferred)
¾	cup crumbled feta cheese
¾	pound cooked shrimp

Mix the vinegar, oil, garlic, pepper, and salt in a small bowl. Combine the lettuce, tomatoes, cucumber, and onion in a large bowl and toss with the dressing. Evenly divide the salad among four serving bowls and top with the olives, cheese, and shrimp.

Per serving: calories 317, protein 25 g, carbohydrates 16 g, fiber 6 g, fat 18 g (monounsaturated 9 g, polyunsaturated 2 g, saturated 6 g), sodium 908 mg

LUNCH

Chef Priscilla's Chicken Satay with Peanut Sauce

Courtesy of Chef Priscilla Willis, Hyatt Huntington Beach, California

Yield: 4 servings

Start to finish: 1 hour, 30 minutes

2	cloves garlic, peeled and minced
1	tablespoon extra virgin olive oil
1	tablespoon low-sodium soy sauce
1	tablespoon lime juice, or lemon juice
½	teaspoon curry powder
¾	pound partially frozen chicken breast, skinless and boneless
8	(10- to 12-inch) bamboo skewers
8	cups chopped lettuce
1	cup sliced cucumber

Peanut Sauce

½	cup coconut milk
4	tablespoons rice wine vinegar
3	tablespoons peanut butter
2	tablespoons lime juice
½	teaspoon chili paste
½	teaspoon ginger root
1	tablespoon xylitol
¼	cup chopped cilantro
¼	teaspoon salt

Mix the garlic, oil, soy sauce, lime juice, and curry powder in a medium bowl. (Put chicken in freezer for 20 minutes if already thawed—this makes it much easier to thinly slice.) Slice the chicken lengthwise into long, thin (1 x 4 x 1/4-inch) slices. Place the chicken in the bowl with the marinade, cover, and refrigerate for at least 1 hour, stirring occasionally.

Soak the bamboo skewers in water for at least 30 minutes. Toss the lettuce and cucumbers in a large bowl and refrigerate.

While the chicken is marinating make the peanut sauce. Combine the coconut milk, vinegar, peanut butter, lime juice, chili paste, ginger root, xylitol, cilantro, and salt in a blender or food processor and process until smooth. Drizzle over chicken skewers.

Thread the chicken slices onto the skewers, working the skewer in and out along the strip. Baste both sides with marinade. Preheat the broiler (or grill or barbeque) to high, and cook the chicken for 2 to 3 minutes on each side, or until golden brown.

To serve, divide lettuce and cucumbers among four serving plates, place 2 chicken skewers on each, and drizzle with peanut sauce.

Per serving: calories 307, protein 25 g, carbohydrates 15 g, fiber 4 g, fat 18 g (monounsaturated 8 g, polyunsaturated 2 g, saturated 8 g), sodium 415 mg

LUNCH

Hot and Sour Soup

As good as you'll find in any Chinese restaurant

Yield: 4 servings
Start to finish: 45 minutes

8	dried shiitake mushrooms or wood-ear mushrooms
3½	cups low-sodium chicken broth
1	cup white mushrooms, juilienned
1½	cups cooked chicken, juilienned
½	cup bamboo shoots, canned, drained, and juilienned
¼	cup carrots, juilienned
3	tablespoons rice vinegar
2	tablespoons low-sodium soy sauce
¼	teaspoon ground black pepper
¼	teaspoon red pepper flakes, or to taste
1	tablespoon cornstarch
3	tablespoons water
1	egg white, lightly beaten
1	teaspoon sesame oil
2	green onions, thinly sliced

Soak the shiitake or wood-ear mushrooms in hot water for 30 minutes, or until soft. Remove the stems and cut into long thin strips. Bring the broth, mushrooms, chicken, bamboo shoots, and carrots to a boil in a large saucepan. Reduce the heat to low and simmer for about 5 minutes. Add the vinegar, soy sauce, black pepper, and red pepper flakes to the soup and cook for another 1 minute.

In a small bowl, dissolve the cornstarch into the water and add to the soup, stirring until it thickens. While stirring, slowly pour the egg white into the soup and cook until the egg turns white. Stir in the sesame oil and top with green onions.

Per serving: calories 289, protein 28 g, carbohydrates 13 g, fiber 2 g, fat 14 g (monounsaturated 6 g, polyunsaturated 3 g, saturated 4 g), sodium 833 mg

Salmon-Avocado Salad
A refreshing change from tuna salad

Yield: 4 servings
Start to finish: 15 minutes

1	(14½-ounce) can salmon
1	stalk celery, diced
⅓	cup diced green bell pepper
2	tablespoons low-fat sour cream
1	tablespoon mayonnaise
1	tablespoon lime juice
½	teaspoon garlic powder
⅛	teaspoon ground black pepper
8	romaine lettuce leaves
2	avocados, halved and seeded
1	large tomato, cut into wedges
½	cucumber, sliced

Drain the salmon and place in a medium mixing bowl. Break into bite-size pieces and remove the bones and skin. Add the celery, green bell pepper, sour cream, mayonnaise, lime juice, garlic powder, and black pepper and gently stir until blended. Arrange lettuce leaves on four salad plates and center an avocado half on each plate of salad greens. Spoon the salmon into the avocados and around the edges. Place tomato wedges and cucumber slices around the avocados.

Per serving: calories 330, protein 24 g, carbohydrates 12 g, fiber 4 g, fat 22 g (monounsaturated 11 g, polyunsaturated 5 g, saturated 4 g), sodium 114 mg

LUNCH

Signature Chef's Salad
A *familiar favorite*

Yield: 4 servings
Start to finish: 10 minutes

12	cups chopped lettuce
¾	cup julienned cooked turkey breast
¾	cup julienned turkey ham
¾	cup julienned reduced-fat cheddar cheese
2	whole eggs, hard-boiled, cut into wedges
2	small tomatoes, cut into wedges
4	tablespoons of ranch dressing (or dressing of your choice)

Place the lettuce in serving bowls. Arrange the turkey, ham, cheese, eggs, and tomatoes on top. Serve with 1 tablespoon salad dressing per person.

Per serving: calories 303, protein 27 g, carbohydrates 11 g, fiber 4 g, fat 17 g (monounsaturated 5 g, polyunsaturated 6 g, saturated 5 g), sodium 810 mg

Heavenly Deviled Eggs
A sinfully delicious snack

Yield: 4 servings
Start to finish: 10 minutes

4	hard-boiled eggs
2	tablespoons mayonnaise
⅓	teaspoon dry mustard
	Pinch salt
	Pinch pepper
	Pinch paprika

SNACKS

Carefully peel eggs and cut in half lengthwise. Remove the yolks and place them in a small bowl. Add the mayonnaise, mustard, salt, and pepper and mix well, mashing the yolks with a fork. Fill the whites with the yolk mixture. Sprinkle with paprika. Cover and refrigerate.

Per serving: calories 107, protein 6 g, carbohydrates 2 g, fiber trace g, fat 8 g (monounsaturated 3 g, polyunsaturated 3 g, saturated 2 g), sodium 148 mg

Raspberry-Lemon Delight
A sugar-free way to satisfy your sweet tooth

Yield: 1 serving
Start to finish: 5 minutes

¼	cup part-skim ricotta cheese
¼	cup raspberries
1	teaspoon lemon juice
¼	teaspoon grated lemon peel
1	drop vanilla extract
4	drops stevia, or Splenda to taste

Mix the ricotta cheese, raspberries, lemon juice, lemon peel, and vanilla extract together in a small bowl, mashing the berries with a fork. Add sweetener to taste.

NOTE: When your sweet tooth starts erupting, experiment with this recipe. We've tried it with unsweetened chocolate, blueberries, coconut and almond extracts, all sweetened with stevia or Splenda. They're all pretty good, but Raspberry-Lemon Delight takes the cake.

Per serving: calories 104, protein 7 g, carbohydrates 7 g, fiber 2 g, fat 7 g (monounsaturated 1 g, polyunsaturated trace g, saturated 3 g), sodium 77 mg

Spicy Salmon with Baby Greens
Dr. Whitaker's personal favorite

Yield: 4 servings
Start to finish: 1 hour, 30 minutes

1	tablespoon xylitol
2	tablespoons chili powder
1	tablespoon onion powder
1	tablespoon garlic powder
1	tablespoon paprika
½	teaspoon salt
¼	teaspoon ground pepper
4	(4-ounce) wild salmon fillets
1	tablespoon plus 2 tablespoons extra virgin olive oil
1	tablespoon balsamic vinegar
2	teaspoons Dijon mustard
1	tablespoon water, if needed
12	cups baby greens

In a small bowl mix together the xylitol, chili powder, onion powder, garlic powder, paprika, salt, and pepper. Set 1½ tablespoons of this spice mixture aside. Rub the remainder on both sides of the salmon fillets. Cover and refrigerate for at least 1 hour.

Mix 1 tablespoon of the olive oil, reserved spices, vinegar, and mustard together in a small bowl. Add a little water to thin, if necessary. Toss the dressing with greens. Divide among four plates.

Preheat the broiler or grill until hot. Rub the salmon with the remaining olive oil and place on the broiler or grill. Cook for 3 to 5 minutes per side, or until just done. Do not overcook. Place salmon on top of each salad and serve.

Per serving: calories 280, protein 26 g, carbohydrates 13 g, fiber 4 g, fat 15 g (monounsaturated 9 g, polyunsaturated 3 g, saturated 2 g), sodium 428 mg

DINNER

"Spaghetti" and Italian Sausage

As close to pasta as you'll get

Yield: 4 servings

Start to finish: 1 hour, 30 minutes

2	cups spaghetti squash (1 small squash, about 1½ pounds)
1	teaspoon extra virgin olive oil
¾	pound Italian turkey sausage, casings removed
½	cup chopped green pepper
½	cup chopped onion
2	cloves garlic, minced
1	(14½ -ounce) can low-sodium tomatoes, chopped, with liquid
½	cup water
¼	cup parsley
1	tablespoon tomato paste
½	teaspoon dried basil
1	tablespoon butter
	Dash salt
	Dash pepper
¼	cup grated Parmesan cheese

Preheat the oven to 375 degrees. Cut the squash in half lengthwise and remove the seeds. Place the squash cut side down in a large baking dish and add enough hot water to completely cover the bottom edges of the squash (about 2 inches of water). Bake for 1 hour or until squash is tender when pierced with a fork. Remove from oven, take squash out of the pan, and cool slightly.

Heat the olive oil in a large skillet. Add the sausage, green pepper, onions, and garlic, and cook, stirring often and breaking up sausage with spoon. Cook for 10 minutes or until sausage is cooked through. Add the tomatoes, water, parsley, tomato paste, and basil and cook for another 10 to 15 minutes, stirring often. Add more water, if necessary.

While the sauce is cooking, scrape the inside of squash with a fork—it will come out in spaghetti-like strands. Add butter, salt, and pepper, and mix well.

To serve, place half a cup of "spaghetti" on each serving plate and top with sauce and a sprinkling of Parmesan cheese.

Per serving: calories 287, protein 22 g, carbohydrates 14 g, fiber 3 g, fat 15 g (monounsaturated 5 g, polyunsaturated 3 g, saturated 5 g), sodium 908 mg

Garlicky Greens
Garlic lovers delight

Yield: 4 servings
Start to finish: 10 minutes

1	pound fresh spinach (about 12 cups)
1	teaspoon extra virgin olive oil
3	cloves garlic, peeled and minced

DINNER

Wash the spinach well and remove the stems. Heat the olive oil over medium heat in a large nonstick skillet. Add the garlic and cook, stirring constantly for 1 minute. Add the spinach to the skillet and continue to cook for 3 or 4 minutes, or until wilted.

Per serving: calories 38, protein 3 g, carbohydrates 5 g, fiber 3 g, fat 2 g (monounsaturated 1 g, polyunsaturated trace, saturated trace), sodium 90 mg

Halibut Dijon

Catch of the day—with a French twist

Yield: 4 servings

Start to finish: 1 hour, 15 minutes

½	cup fresh lemon juice
1	tablespoon lemon peel, minced
¼	cup Dijon mustard
2	tablespoons tarragon, finely chopped (or 2 teaspoons dried tarragon)
2	tablespoons parsley, finely chopped
2	tablespoons green onions, finely chopped
2	tablespoons extra virgin olive oil
½	teaspoon ground pepper
¼	teaspoon salt
4	(4-ounce) halibut fillets or steaks
	Tarragon or parsley sprigs for garnish

DINNER

In a bowl mix together the lemon juice, peel, mustard, tarragon, parsley, green onions, olive oil, pepper, and salt. Place the halibut in a shallow baking dish and pour the marinade over the fish. Turn the fish to coat evenly. Cover and refrigerate for at least 1 hour.

Preheat the grill or broiler. Remove the fish from the marinade and cook about 3 inches from the grill or broiler for 3 to 6 minutes on each side, depending on thickness, or until opaque. Garnish with sprigs of tarragon or parsley.

Per serving: calories 214, protein 25 g, carbohydrates 6 g, fiber 1 g, fat 10 g (monounsaturated 6 g, polyunsaturated 2 g, saturated 1 g), sodium 386 mg

Shrimp Shish Kabobs

A savory seafood dish perfect for the grill or broiler

Yield: 4 servings
Start to finish: 45 minutes

3	tablespoons lemon juice
1	tablespoon extra virgin olive oil
1	tablespoon low-sodium soy sauce
¼	teaspoon ground black pepper
⅛	teaspoon red pepper flakes
1	pound large shrimp (about 25), cleaned, peeled, and deveined, tails on
4	(10 to 12-inch) bamboo skewers

Combine the lemon juice, olive oil, soy sauce, pepper, and red pepper flakes in a medium bowl. Add the shrimp, stir to coat shrimp, and refrigerate for at least 30 minutes, stirring occasionally.

Soak the bamboo skewers in water for 30 minutes while the shrimp marinates. Remove from the marinade and thread the shrimp onto the skewers, leaving a little room between to ensure even cooking.

Preheat grill or broiler. Cook skewers for 2 to 4 minutes per side, just until the shrimp turn pink.

Per serving: calories 156, protein 23 g, carbohydrates 2 g, fiber trace, fat 5 g (monounsaturated 3 g, polyunsaturated 1 g, saturated 1 g), sodium 318 mg

DINNER

Southwestern Chicken Fajitas
A *healthy south-of-the-border favorite*

Yield: 4 servings
Start to finish: 20 minutes

¼	cup lime juice
2	cloves garlic, peeled and minced
1	teaspoon coriander
1	teaspoon cumin
¼	teaspoon red pepper flakes
¾	pound boneless, skinless chicken breast, cut into 1½ x 1-inch strips
	Olive oil spray
1	medium onion, sliced lengthwise
1	large green bell pepper (or mixture of red and green peppers), cut into strips
½	cup grated reduced-fat cheddar cheese
½	cup salsa
8	romaine lettuce leaves

In a large glass or porcelain bowl combine the lime juice, garlic, coriander, cumin, and red pepper flakes. Mix well and add the chicken strips, stir, cover, and refrigerate for at least 1 hour.

Heat a large nonstick skillet over medium-high heat. Spray with olive oil. Add the chicken to the skillet and cook, stirring frequently, for 3 to 4 minutes, or until done. Remove from the skillet. Add the onion and green bell pepper to the skillet and cook, stirring often, until crisp-tender, about 5 minutes. Return the chicken to the pan and cook for 1 to 2 minutes, or until heated through.

Spoon the chicken mixture onto lettuce leaves. Top with cheese, salsa, and guacamole (recipe on next page).

Per serving: calories 164, protein 24 g, carbohydrates 9 g, fiber 2 g, fat 4 g (monounsaturated 1 g, polyunsaturated 1 g, saturated 1 g), sodium 267 mg

DINNER

Gringo Guacamole
A perfect companion for fajitas

Yield: 4 servings
Start to finish: 15 minutes

1	large ripe avocado
1	tablespoon lime or lemon juice
¼	teaspoon salt
¼	cup chopped tomato
2	teaspoons chopped onion
1	tablespoon chopped cilantro (optional)

In a medium bowl mash the avocado with a fork until smooth. Add the lime juice, salt, tomato, onion, and cilantro, if using, and stir until blended. Serve with Southwestern Chicken Fajitas.

Per serving: calories 86, protein 1 g, carbohydrates 5 g, fiber 1 g, fat 8 g (monounsaturated 5 g, polyunsaturated 1 g, saturated 1 g), sodium 140 mg

DINNER

Green Beans Extraordinaire

Not your mama's green beans

Yield: 4 servings

Start to finish: 20 minutes

2	teaspoons extra virgin olive oil
1	onion, chopped
3	cloves garlic, peeled and minced
1	pound fresh green beans (trimmed)
½	teaspoon salt
¼	cup water

Heat the olive oil in a large, covered skillet over medium heat. Add the onion and garlic and sauté for two minutes. Add the beans, salt, and water and stir well. Reduce the heat to low, cover, and steam for 10 to 15 minutes, or until just tender. If any liquid remains, turn up heat and boil off before serving.

Per serving: calories 65, protein 2 g, carbohydrates 10 g, fiber 4 g, fat 2 g (monounsaturated 2 g, polyunsaturated trace, saturated 0 g), sodium 274 mg

DINNER

Easy Baked Salmon
Chockfull of heart-healthy omega-3 fats

Yield: 4 servings
Start to finish: 30 minutes

2	teaspoons extra virgin olive oil
2	tablespoons lemon juice
1½	tablespoons chives, fresh or freeze-dried
1	teaspoon grated lemon peel
¼	teaspoon salt
⅛	teaspoon ground black pepper
	Olive oil spray
4	(4-ounce) wild salmon fillets

Preheat the oven to 400 degrees. Combine the olive oil, lemon juice, chives, lemon peel, salt, and pepper in a small bowl and stir until well blended. Spray a large, shallow baking pan with olive oil. Place the salmon fillets skin side down in the dish and rub the oil mixture over the fish. Bake for 12 to 15 minutes, or until just done. (Do not overcook.)

Per serving: calories 154, protein 23 g, carbohydrates 1 g, fiber trace g, fat 6 g (monounsaturated 3 g, polyunsaturated 2 g, saturated 1 g), sodium 209 mg

DINNER

Steamed Broccoli with Lemon Sauce

Say goodbye to boring broccoli

Yield: 4 servings

Start to finish: 20 minutes

½	cup low-sodium chicken broth
2	tablespoons lemon juice
2	teaspoons cornstarch
½	teaspoon low-sodium soy sauce
¼	teaspoon xylitol
1	teaspoon butter
4	cups broccoli florets

In a small saucepan over medium-low heat, combine the chicken broth, lemon juice, cornstarch, soy sauce, and xylitol. Stir until the cornstarch is dissolved. Increase the heat to medium and bring to a boil , stirring constantly. Reduce the heat to low and cook for another 3 to 5 minutes, stirring constantly, or until the sauce is thick. Add the butter. Keep warm.

Steam the broccoli over boiling water for 5 to 7 minutes, or until just tender. (Or place in a covered glass dish with 2 tablespoons of water and cook in the microwave for 2 to 3 minutes.) Drain the broccoli and serve with lemon sauce.

Per serving: calories 67, protein 4 g, carbohydrates 10 g, fiber 4 g, fat 2 g (monounsaturated 1 g, polyunsaturated trace, saturated 1 g), sodium 84 mg

Bayside Broiled Chicken

Moist, tangy, and full of flavor

Yield: 4 servings

Start to finish: 1 hour, 30 minutes

8	bone-in chicken thighs (about 3½ pounds), skin removed, trimmed
1	tablespoon lime juice
1	cup plain, low-fat yogurt
2	garlic cloves, peeled and minced
1	tablespoon fresh ginger, minced
2	teaspoons paprika
½	teaspoon salt

Place the chicken in a large bowl and coat with the lime juice. In a separate small bowl, mix the yogurt, garlic, ginger, paprika, and salt. Pour over the chicken and stir to coat. Cover and refrigerate for at least 1 hour. (You may marinate for up to 24 hours.)

Preheat the broiler and position the rack in the upper third of the oven. Remove the chicken from the bowl and dispose of the excess marinade. Place the chicken on the broiler rack and broil for 15 minutes, turning once or twice, or until browned on top. Set the oven to 400 degrees and cook about 15 minutes longer, or until the chicken is juicy and cooked through. (Thigh meat remains a dark pink color, even when thoroughly cooked.) Serve immediately.

Per serving: calories 213, protein 31 g, carbohydrates 6 g, fiber 0 g, fat 6 g (monounsaturated 2 g, polyunsaturated 1 g, saturated 2 g), sodium 429 mg

DINNER

Lemon Pepper Asparagus

Give asparagus a flavorful boost

Yield: 4 servings
Start to finish: 15 minutes

1	pound asparagus, washed and trimmed
1	teaspoon lemon juice
	Dash ground black pepper
	Dash lemon pepper
	Dash garlic powder
	Dash seasoned salt

Steam the asparagus over boiling water for 5 to 7 minutes, or until just tender. (Or place in a covered glass dish with 2 tablespoons of water and cook in the microwave for 2 to 3 minutes.) Place on a serving dish and drizzle with lemon juice. Sprinkle pepper, lemon pepper, garlic powder, and seasoned salt on top to taste.

Per serving: calories 15, protein 1 g, carbohydrates 3 g, fiber 1 g, fat 0 g, sodium 55 mg

DINNER

Seared Ahi Salad with Wasabi Dressing
A delicious Asian main-dish salad

Yield: 4 servings
Start to finish: 15 minutes

3	tablespoons extra virgin olive oil
2	tablespoons low-sodium soy sauce
2	tablespoons rice vinegar
1	teaspoon wasabi paste
12	cups mixed baby lettuce
8	radishes, sliced
1	cucumber, thinly sliced
2	tablespoons five-spice powder
½	teaspoon salt
1	teaspoon coarsely ground black pepper
4	(3-ounce) Ahi (tuna) steaks
	Olive oil spray

DINNER

Combine the olive oil, soy sauce, rice vinegar, and wasabi paste in a small bowl and mix well. (You may add more or less wasabi to taste.) Toss the lettuce, radishes, and cucumber in a bowl. Mix the five-spice powder, salt, and pepper together and coat the tuna steaks evenly. Heat a grill or skillet over high heat and spray with olive oil. Add the tuna steaks and sear for 2 minutes on each side. Remove from the pan and thinly slice on an angle. Toss the salad with the dressing, arrange on four plates, and place an Ahi steak on top of each salad.

Per serving: calories 261, protein 23 g, carbohydrates 10 g, fiber 4 g, fat 15 g (monounsaturated 9 g, polyunsaturated 3 g, saturated 3 g), sodium 352 mg

Salmon Patties on Field Greens

A seafood salad everyone is sure to love

Yield: 4 servings
Start to finish: 1 hour, 15 minutes

1	(14¾-ounce) can salmon, well drained
1	egg, lightly beaten
⅓	cup finely chopped onion
⅓	cup finely chopped celery
¼	cup mayonnaise
2	tablespoons oat bran
1	tablespoon Mrs. Dash (salt-free seasoning)
¼	teaspoon ground black pepper
	Dash Tabasco sauce
	Olive oil spray

Dressing

¼	cup light mayonnaise
¼	cup chopped dill pickles
¼	cup chopped green onions
2	tablespoons lemon juice
1	to 2 tablespoons water
¼	teaspoon pepper
12	cups mixed field greens (or lettuce of your choice), torn into bite-sized pieces

In a medium bowl, break the salmon into flakes, discarding the bones and skin and taking care not to break salmon up too much. Pat dry with paper towels. In another bowl, stir together the egg, onion, celery, mayonnaise, oat bran, Mrs. Dash, black pepper, and Tabasco sauce until well blended. Gently fold into the salmon. Cover and refrigerate for at least 45 minutes.

Prepare dressing by combining the mayonnaise, pickles, green onions, lemon juice, water, and pepper in a small bowl. Stir well, adding more or less water to achieve desired thickness, and refrigerate.

Heat a large nonstick skillet over medium heat. Spray with olive oil spray. Measure ¼ cup salmon mixture and form into a flat patty. Repeat with the remaining salmon. Cook the salmon cakes, four at a time, in hot skillet for 2 to 3 minutes, flattening somewhat with a spatula. Turn carefully and cook for another 2 to 3 minutes, or until golden brown. Gently remove from the skillet. Cook the remaining salmon patties. (Handle the salmon patties gingerly—they're somewhat fragile.)

To serve, divide the field greens among four plates, top each with 2 salmon cakes, and spoon dressing over top.

Per serving: calories 321, protein 26 g, carbohydrates 14 g, fiber 4 g, fat 20 g (monounsaturated 5 g, polyunsaturated 9 g, saturated 3 g), sodium 377 mg

DINNER

Joe's Special

There's nothing average about this Joe

- Yield: 4 servings

Start to finish: 20 minutes

1	teaspoon extra virgin olive oil
¾	pound lean ground turkey
2	medium onions, finely chopped
2	cloves garlic, peeled and finely minced
½	pound mushrooms, sliced
	Dash Tabasco sauce
¼	teaspoon salt
¼	teaspoon ground black pepper
¼	teaspoon dried oregano
1	(10-ounce) package fresh spinach, chopped
2	whole eggs
¼	cup Parmesan cheese

DINNER

Heat the oil in a large skilled over medium-high heat. Add the ground turkey and stir often, breaking up chunks, until brown. Drain excess fat. Add the onions, garlic, and mushrooms to the skillet and reduce the heat to medium. Continue cooking, stirring often, until the onions are tender, about 5 minutes. Stir in the Tabasco, salt, pepper, oregano, and spinach and cook for another 3 to 4 minutes, or until the spinach has wilted. Beat the eggs in a small bowl and add to the skillet. Cook, stirring, until eggs are set. Stir in the cheese.

Per serving: calories 248, protein 23 g, carbohydrates 10 g, fiber 4 g, fat 12 g (monounsaturated 5 g, polyunsaturated 2 g, saturated 4 g), sodium 395 mg

Bayou Shrimp

A Creole creation your family will love

Yield: 4 servings
Start to finish: 30 minutes

1	teaspoon extra virgin olive oil
1	whole onion, cut into 1-inch pieces
½	large green bell pepper, cut into 1-inch pieces
½	large red bell pepper, cut into 1-inch pieces
3	cloves garlic, peeled and minced
1	pound shrimp, large or medium, peeled, deveined, with tails removed
1	(14½-ounce) can low-sodium tomatoes, chopped, with juice
1	teaspoon chopped fresh thyme or ¼ teaspoon dried thyme
½	teaspoon ground black pepper
¼	teaspoon seasoned salt
⅛	teaspoon red pepper flakes

DINNER

In a large nonstick skillet, heat the olive oil over medium-high heat. Add the onion, bell peppers, and garlic and cook for 3 or 4 minutes, stirring occasionally, or until crisp-tender. Add the shrimp to the skillet along with tomatoes (including their juice), thyme, black pepper, seasoned salt, and red pepper flakes. Bring to a boil, reduce the heat, cover and simmer for 3 to 4 minutes, stirring occasionally, or until shrimp are pink and firm.

Per serving: calories 159, protein 24 g, carbohydrates 7 g, fiber 1 g, fat 3 g (monounsaturated 1 g, polyunsaturated 1 g, saturated trace), sodium 258 mg

Broccoli-Olive Salad

Bursting with cancer-fighting phytonutrients

Yield: 4 servings
Start to finish: 40 minutes

2	tablespoons extra virgin olive oil
2	tablespoons balsamic vinegar
¼	teaspoon seasoned salt
⅛	teaspoon black pepper
3	cups coarsely chopped broccoli florets
2	tablespoons finely chopped onion
2	tablespoons sliced black olives

In a small bowl, mix together the oil, vinegar, salt, and pepper. In a medium bowl, combine the broccoli, onion, and olives and toss with the dressing. Let marinate 30 minutes to 1 hour before serving.

Per serving: calories 84, protein 2 g, carbohydrates 4 g, fiber 2 g, fat 7 g (monounsaturated 5 g, polyunsaturated 1 g, saturated 1 g), sodium 137 mg

DINNER

Pacific Pork Carnitas

A do-ahead slow cooker recipe that's sure to please a crowd

Yield: 20 servings
Start to finish: 9 hours

5	pounds pork tenderloin, lean, boneless
1	large red onion, chopped
1	(3½-ounce) can green chile peppers, with juice
2	cups salsa verde (green salsa)
12	ounces beer (Pacifico or other Mexican beer preferred)
40	romaine lettuce leaves
1	cup chopped cilantro
3	cups shredded low-fat cheddar cheese
1½	cups nonfat sour cream

Cut the pork tenderloin in half and place in a slow cooker. Combine the onion, green chiles, salsa, and beer. Add three-quarters of the onion mixture to the slow cooker, cover, and cook on low for 7 to 8 hours.

Using a fork or tongs, gently pull the pork apart. Cover and let cook another 1 to 2 hours, or until pork is cooked through.

Place 2 lettuce leaves on each plate and fill each with a scoop of the pork. Divide the remaining onion mixture evenly onto the meat and garnish with cilantro, cheese, and a dollop of sour cream.

Per serving: calories 198, protein 27 g, carbohydrates 7 g, fiber 1 g, fat 6 g (monounsaturated 3 g, polyunsaturated 1 g, saturated 2 g), sodium 241 mg

DINNER

Wilted Greens

Loaded with vitamin A and other nutrients

Yield: 4 servings
Start to finish: 40 minutes

1	pound greens (mustard, turnip, collards, or a mixture)
1	clove garlic, peeled and minced
1	medium onion, chopped
2	cups chicken broth
½	teaspoon ground black pepper

Wash the greens carefully and remove any tough stems. Place the greens, garlic, onion, broth, and black pepper in a large saucepan or stockpot. Bring to a boil over medium heat. Reduce the heat and cook, stirring occasionally, for 30 minutes, or until tender. Drain and serve.

Per serving: calories 61, protein 6 g, carbohydrates 9 g, fiber 4 g, fat 1 g (monounsaturated trace, polyunsaturated trace, saturated trace), sodium 288 mg

DINNER

Teriyaki Chicken with Mushroom Gravy

"I come from a family where gravy is considered a beverage," Erma Bombeck

Yield: 4 servings
Start to finish: 1 hour, 15 minutes

1	teaspoon extra virgin olive oil
4	(4-ounce) chicken breasts, boneless, skinless
1	cup sliced mushrooms
¾	cup water
½	cup low-sodium chicken broth
2	tablespoons low-sodium soy sauce
1	teaspoon rice vinegar
1	teaspoon ginger, grated or ½ teaspoon dried ginger
1	clove garlic, minced
1	tablespoon cornstarch
¼	cup cold water

DINNER

Preheat the oven to 350 degrees. In a large, nonstick skillet, heat the olive oil and brown the chicken breasts for about 2 minutes per side. Place the chicken in a baking dish and bake for 45 minutes.

In a medium saucepan combine the mushrooms, water, chicken broth, soy sauce, vinegar, ginger, and garlic. Bring to a boil. Reduce the heat to low. Stir the cornstarch into the cold water until dissolved. Add to the saucepan and cook for another 1 minute, stirring constantly, or until the gravy thickens. Pour the gravy over the chicken.

NOTE: This recipe goes great with the Whitaker Wellness Mashed "Potatoes" on page 217.

Per serving: calories 249, protein 24 g, carbohydrates 4 g, fiber trace, fat 15 g (monounsaturated 7 g, polyunsaturated 1 g, saturated 6 g), sodium 425 mg

Sole a l'Orange

Citrus and seafood: a perfect combo

Yield: 4 servings

Start to finish: 30 minutes

1	orange, juiced (about ½ cup)
1	tablespoon low-sodium soy sauce
1	tablespoon fresh ginger root, grated
4	(4-ounce) sole fillets
1	plus 1 teaspoon extra virgin olive oil
1	pound snow pea pods, trimmed

Combine the orange juice, soy sauce, and ginger in a shallow pan. Add sole fillets, turn to coat, cover, and refrigerate for 15 to 20 minutes.

Heat 1 teaspoon of the olive oil in a large nonstick skillet over medium-high heat. Remove the sole from the marinade (reserve the marinade) and cook in the skillet until just firm and opaque, about 3 minutes per side. Remove the sole from the skillet and keep warm. Add the remaining olive oil. Place the snow peas in the skillet and stir-fry for 1 to 2 minutes. Remove peas and keep warm. Pour the reserved marinade into the skillet, bring to a boil, and cook for 1 to 2 minutes. Pour the sauce over the sole before serving.

Per serving: calories 190, protein 25 g, carbohydrates 13 g, fiber 4 g, fat 4 g (monounsaturated 2 g, polyunsaturated 1 g, saturated 1 g), sodium 247 mg

Spinach-Cheese Stuffed Chicken Breasts

An elegant dish that's sure to wow your guests

Yield: 4 servings
Start to finish: 1 hour, 15 minutes

1	teaspoon extra virgin olive oil
1	medium onion, finely chopped
¼	teaspoon salt
¼	teaspoon ground black pepper
1	(10-ounce) bag fresh spinach, washed, stemmed, and chopped
½	cup reduced-fat ricotta cheese
½	cup grated Parmesan cheese
	Olive oil spray
4	(3-ounce) skinless, boneless chicken breasts

Preheat the oven to 350 degrees. Heat the olive oil in a medium, nonstick skillet over medium heat. Add the onion, salt, and pepper and sauté for 5 minutes. Add the spinach and cook for another 4 minutes, or until spinach is wilted and all the moisture is evaporated. Place in a medium bowl and let cool. Add the cheeses and mix well. Spray a medium baking dish with olive oil. Slice the chicken breasts lengthwise, creating a pocket in each. (Be sure to leave top, bottom, and one side intact.) Divide the cheese mixture evenly and stuff into each pocket. Place the chicken in a baking dish and bake for 45 minutes, or until chicken is cooked through.

Per serving: calories 225, protein 29 g, carbohydrates 7 g, fiber 2 g, fat 9 g (monounsaturated 3 g, polyunsaturated 1 g, saturated 4 g), sodium 460 mg

DINNER

Shrimp and Broccoli Stir-Fry

An Asian sensation swimming with flavor

Yield: 4 servings
Start to finish: 20 minutes

1	tablespoon extra virgin olive oil
1	pound shrimp, large, peeled, deveined, with tails removed
¼	cup water
1¼	pound broccoli florets, broken into bite-sized pieces
1½	tablespoons chili-garlic sauce
1	(8-ounce) can bamboo shoots (optional)

Heat a large nonstick skillet over high heat until hot and add the oil, swirling to coat. Add the shrimp and cook 1½ to 2 minutes, stirring constantly, or until just slightly undercooked. Remove from the heat and set aside. Add ¼ cup water and broccoli to the hot skillet. Cover and steam approximately 2 minutes, or until just tender. Pour off the excess water, if any remains.

Return the shrimp to the skillet, along with chili-garlic sauce and bamboo shoots and stir-fry until all ingredients are coated in sauce and piping hot. Serve immediately.

Per serving: calories 207, protein 28 g, carbohydrates 11 g, fiber 6 g, fat 6 g (monounsaturated 3 g, polyunsaturated 1 g, saturated 1 g), sodium 209 mg

DINNER

Roasted Chicken
A classic recipe for any occasion

Yield: 12 servings
Start to finish: 1 hour, 45 minutes

6	pounds roasting chicken
1	teaspoon extra virgin olive oil
½	teaspoon salt
½	teaspoon ground black pepper

Preheat the oven to 425 degrees. Place a rack in a roasting pan or large baking dish. Rinse the chicken well inside and out; dry with paper towels. Rub the chicken with olive oil, sprinkle with salt and pepper, and place in the prepared pan, breast side up. Cook for 75 to 90 minutes, or until a thermometer inserted in the thigh or breast registers 170 degrees. You may baste if desired, but it isn't necessary. If the drippings in the pan begin to smoke, remove them with a spoon and add a little water. Drain the juices from cavity of chicken.

NOTE: Remove the skin before eating to dramatically reduce fat. Nutritional analysis below is with skin. If you remove the skin, fat content drops down to about 8 grams.

Per serving: calories 357, protein 28 g, carbohydrates 0 g, fiber 0 g, fat 26 g (monounsaturated 11 g, polyunsaturated 6 g, saturated 7 g), sodium 200 mg

DINNER

Zucchini Parmesan Sauté

Parmesan cheese elevates zucchini to new heights

Yield: 4 servings
Start to finish: 15 minutes

1	teaspoon extra virgin olive oil
6	cups thinly sliced zucchini
¼	teaspoon pepper
¼	cup grated Parmesan cheese

Heat the olive oil over medium-high heat in a large nonstick skillet. Add the zucchini and cook, stirring frequently until just tender, about 5 minutes. Remove from the heat, sprinkle with pepper, and stir in the Parmesan cheese.

Per serving: calories 57, protein 4 g, carbohydrates 5 g, fiber 2 g, fat 3 g (monounsaturated 1 g, polyunsaturated trace, saturated 1 g), sodium 98 mg

DINNER

Cashew Chicken
An easy stir-fry that's sure to satisfy

Yield: 4 servings
Start to finish: 15 minutes

½	cup low-sodium chicken broth
2	tablespoons low-sodium soy sauce
1	clove garlic, minced
1	teaspoon grated fresh ginger, or ½ teaspoon dried, ground ginger
1	tablespoon cornstarch
2	teaspoons extra virgin olive oil (divided use)
¾	pound boneless, skinless chicken breast, cut into half-inch cubes
1	onion, cut in half-inch cubes
½	green bell pepper, cut in half-inch cubes
½	red bell pepper, cut in half-inch cubes
⅓	cup cashews

Combine the chicken broth, soy sauce, garlic, and ginger in a small bowl and stir to mix. Add the cornstarch and stir well. Set aside.

Heat 1 teaspoon of olive oil in a large nonstick skillet or wok over medium-high heat. Add the chicken and cook, stirring until cooked through, about 3 minutes. Remove and set aside.

Add the remaining oil to the pan, followed by the onion and peppers. Cook for 3 to 4 minutes, stirring often, or until vegetables are tender but crisp. Return the chicken to the pan, and cook for 1 minute. Add the sauce and cook, stirring constantly for 1 to 2 minutes, or until the sauce is thick. Stir in the cashews and serve immediately.

Per serving: calories 221, protein 23 g, carbohydrates 10 g, fiber 2 g, fat 10 g (monounsaturated 6 g, polyunsaturated 2 g, saturated 2 g), sodium 413 mg

DINNER

Poached Salmon with Cucumber Sauce

An easy way to get your catch of the day

Yield: 4 servings
Start to finish: 30 minutes

Cucumber Sauce

1	cup cucumber, drained and finely diced
½	cup low-fat or nonfat sour cream
¼	teaspoon celery salt
¼	teaspoon ground black pepper

Salmon

2	cups water, boiling
2	chicken bouillon cubes (low-sodium preferred)
1	tablespoon white vinegar
1	small onion, sliced
1	teaspoon dill weed
¼	teaspoon ground black pepper
4	(4-ounce) salmon steaks (about 1 inch thick)

To make the cucumber sauce, in a small bowl mix together the cucumber, sour cream, celery salt, and black pepper.

In a large skillet over high heat combine the water, bouillon, vinegar, onion, dill weed, and black pepper. Reduce the heat to low. Cover and simmer for 5 minutes. Add the salmon. Cover and simmer for 8 minutes, or until the fish flakes easily. Spoon the cucumber sauce evenly over the salmon and serve immediately.

Per serving: calories 149, protein 23 g, carbohydrates 3 g, fiber 1 g, fat 4 g (monounsaturated 1 g, polyunsaturated 2 g, saturated 1 g), sodium 449 mg

Whitaker Wellness Mashed "Potatoes"
Almost as good as the real thing

Yield: 4 servings
Start to finish: 15 minutes

8	cups cauliflower florets
⅓	cup half-and-half
2	tablespoons butter
1	clove garlic, peeled and minced
¼	teaspoon salt
⅛	teaspoon ground black pepper

Cook the cauliflower in a steamer (or in a microwave in a covered dish with 3 tablespoons water) until tender, about 10 minutes. Do not overcook. Drain well. Combine the cauliflower, half-and-half, butter, garlic, salt, and pepper in a food processor. Pulse until smooth.

Per serving: calories 128, protein 5 g, carbohydrates 11 g, fiber 5 g, fat 8 g (monounsaturated 2 g, polyunsaturated trace, saturated 5 g), sodium 260 mg

DINNER

Lettuce Wrapped Tacos

Tasty tacos minus the tortillas

Yield: 4 servings
Start to finish: 20 minutes

	Olive oil spray
¾	pound lean ground turkey
1	small red onion, chopped
¼	cup water
½	package of low-sodium taco seasoning
8	romaine lettuce leaves
1	tomato, chopped
1	avocado, cut into strips
¾	cup low-fat cheddar cheese, shredded
½	cup salsa

Spray a large, nonstick skillet with olive oil and add the turkey and half of the onion. Cook on medium-high, stirring constantly, until the turkey is browned. Add the water and taco seasoning and continue cooking for another 1 to 2 minutes, or until the seasoning is evenly distributed. Place 2 lettuce leaves on each plate and spoon the taco mixture on top. Evenly distribute the remaining onion, tomato, and avocado and garnish with the cheese and salsa.

Per serving: calories 291, protein 23 g, carbohydrates 14 g, fiber 3 g, fat 16 g (monounsaturated 8 g, polyunsaturated 2 g, saturated 4 g), sodium 633 mg

DINNER

OVERVIEW OF NUTRITIONAL SUPPLEMENTS FOR WEIGHT LOSS

SUPPLEMENT	ACTIONS	DOSAGE	SAFETY INFO	COMMENTS
5-HTP	Helps balance levels of serotonin, a neurotransmitter that affects appetite	50–100 mg one to three times a day between meals	Do not take with antidepressants, tramadol, caridopa, or triptin drugs; high doses may cause nausea or diarrhea.	Most helpful in cutting carbohydrate cravings; also promotes sleep when taken at bedtime.
Alpha lipoic acid	Improves insulin sensitivity and suppresses appetite	100–200 mg twice a day	Safe and well tolerated; may lower blood sugar, so diabetics should monitor blood sugar levels.	A potent antioxidant that is highly therapeutic for diabetes and diabetic complications.
Bitter orange (*Citrus aurantium*)	Increases metabolism and thermogenesis	100–200 mg one to three times a day, between meals; look for a standardized extract and take no more than 20 mg of synephrine, the active ingredient, per dose	A stimulant that may raise blood pressure and heart rate, alter heart rhythm, and cause anxiety and insomnia in some people. Should not be taken by people with significant diseases or those taking certain prescription and over-the-counter drugs. Do not take for prolonged periods.	Often taken in combination with caffeine; discontinue at once if side effects are noted. Taking late in the day may interfere with sleep.
Caffeine	Increases metabolism and burns calories	100–200 mg one to three times a day	High doses may cause nervousness and insomnia.	Drinking coffee or other caffeinated beverages is another option; a large cup of coffee contains about 100 mg of caffeine.
Chitosan	Blocks fat absorption in intestines	1,000–2,000 mg twice a day, before or after meals	May bind to and remove fat-soluble nutrients.	Do not recommend.
Chromium	Improves insulin sensitivity	200 mcg two or three times daily, with meals	Doses above 1,500 mcg may be toxic.	Most useful for those with abdominal obesity and other signs of insulin resistance.
CLA	Helps increase muscle mass while promoting fat loss; particularly effective on abdominal fat	3 g per day, 1 g with each meal	Generally well tolerated, but large doses may cause GI upset; may worsen blood sugar control, so diabetics should use with caution.	Recommended for excess abdominal fat. Tonalin is the best-studied brand.

OVERVIEW OF NUTRITIONAL SUPPLEMENTS FOR WEIGHT LOSS

SUPPLEMENT	ACTIONS	DOSAGE	SAFETY INFO	COMMENTS
DHEA	Improves insulin sensitivity and helps reduce abdominal fat	Average starting doses are 25 mg per day for women, 50 mg for men	Large doses may causes adrogenic effects in women.	Recommended only for people over 45; blood levels should be checked to confirm correct dose. Provides additional benefits for older men and women.
EGCG	Increases thermogenesis and suppresses appetite	Depends on concentration of green tea extract; use as directed.	Safe and well tolerated.	Green tea and ECGC have a plethora of health benefits.
Ephedra	Increases metabolism and burns calories	10 mg one to three times a day	A stimulant that may raise blood pressure and heart rate, alter heart rhythm, and cause anxiety and insomnia in some people. Should not be taken for prolonged periods or by those with significant diseases or taking certain drugs.	Currently not available.
Fish Oil	Improves glucose and fat metabolism	2 capsules per day (320 mg EPA, 320 mg DHA)	Very safe and well tolerated.	Recommended for everyone.
Glucomannan	Provides fiber and reduces appetite	½ teaspoon in 8-ounces of water 30 minutes to an hour before meals.	May cause gas and bloating; build up to recommended dose gradually.	Also improves constipation and blood sugar control.
Garcinia cambogia (HCA)	Suppresses appetite and increases thermogenesis	250 mg three times a day with meals	Safe and well tolerated.	Conflicting results, but observable effects.
Hoodia gordonii	Reduces appetite	3,000-4,000 mg of powdered herb	Appears to be safe and effective, but research is in early stages.	Quality of some supplements questionable; buy only from established manufacturers.
Multivitamin & mineral supplement	Multiple actions	See page 103	Very safe. Large doses of vitamin C and magnesium may cause gastrointestinal upset.	Everyone should take a good multivitamin.
Phaseolus vulgaris	Blocks starches and carbohydrates	500-1,000 mg before meals	Concern about safety of undigested carbohydrates in GI tract.	Do not recommend.
Pyruvate	Increases metabolic rate	20+ g per day in divided doses	Usually recommended in smaller doses, which is not supported by research.	Recommend only in larger doses.

RESOURCES

THE WHITAKER WELLNESS WEIGHT LOSS PROGRAM WEBSITE

WWW.WHITAKERWEIGHTLOSS.COM

Let us help you achieve your weight loss goals by visiting our website, where you'll find:

- Help in setting realistic weight loss goals
- Commitment contracts, exercise logs, and food diaries to download and print out
- Regular e-mail reminders and motivational tips to help you stay on track
- New recipes and suggestions for dining out
- Additional exercises and fitness tips

DR. WHITAKER'S MONTHLY NEWSLETTER HEALTH & HEALING

Since 1991, Dr. Whitaker's monthly newsletter *Health & Healing* has reached millions of readers, providing them with safe, natural solutions to a multitude of health problems. *Health & Healing* has been rated by *Time* magazine as one of the top ten health newsletters in the country. To subscribe:

Health & Healing
www.drwhitaker.com
(800) 539-8219

NUTRITIONAL SUPPLEMENTS

For the past 20 years, Dr. Whitaker has formulated a complete line of nutritional supplements. For more information or to request a catalog:

> Forward Nutrition
> *www.drwhitaker.com*
> (800) 722-8008

The nutritional supplements discussed in this book are widely available in health food stores and some drugstores. They may also be purchased online.

THE WHITAKER WELLNESS INSTITUTE

Founded by Julian Whitaker, M.D., the Whitaker Wellness Institute in Newport Beach, California, is one of the oldest and most comprehensive alternative medicine clinics in the United States. Since 1979, more than 40,000 patients with heart disease, diabetes, obesity, and other serious diseases have come to the clinic seeking treatment with safe, proven therapies that are ignored by conventional physicians.

Patients participate in the clinic's one-, two-, or three-week Back to Health Program, which involves extensive medical evaluation, diagnostic testing, and treatment. They receive a personalized nutritional supplement prescription, an individualized exercise program, and a therapeutic diet, and they undergo treatment with the unique therapies offered at Whitaker Wellness.

During their stay at the clinic, patients also attend lectures by our physicians and informative, hands-on nutrition and cooking workshops. They participate in exercise and stress management classes and eat delicious, healthful meals prepared by our gourmet chef. They also enjoy the support and guidance of our caring, professional staff, as well as the encouragement and camaraderie of their fellow patients. To learn more about the clinic:

> Whitaker Wellness Institute
> 4321 Birch Street
> Newport Beach, CA 92660
> (800) 488-1500
> *www.whitakerwellness.com*

NOTES

PREFACE

1. S. J. Olshansky and others, "A Potential Decline in Life Expectancy in the 21st Century," New England Journal of Medicine (2005): 352 (11):1138–44.

CHAPTER 1

1. D. T. Felson, "Weight and Osteoarthritis," *Journal of Rheumatology,* (1995): 43:7–9.

2. J. Anderson and others, "Factors Associated with Osteoarthritis of the Knee in the First National Health and Nutrition Examination (HANES I)," *American Journal of Epidemiology,* (1988): 128:179–189.

3. E. E. Calle and others, "Overweight, Obesity, and Mortality from Cancer in a Prospectively Studied Cohort of U.S. Adults, *New England Journal of Medicine* (2003): 345(17):1625–1638.

CHAPTER 3

1. Center for Disease Control (CDC), "Overweight and Obesity: Frequently Asked Questions (FAQs),. Oct 6, 2004, http://www.cdc.gov/nccdphp/dnpa/obesity/faq.htm.

2. ———, Health and Human Services News, "Obesity Still on the Rise, New Data Show," Oct 8, 2002, http://www.cdc.gov/nchs/pressroom/02news/obesityonrise.htm.

3. ———, "Health, United States, 2004," 175–6 (table 69), http://www.cdc.gov/nchs/data/hus/hus04trend.pdf#069.

4. ———, National Center for Health Statistics, "Overweight and Obesity by Age: United States 1960–2002," Health United States, 2004, http://www.cdc.gov/nchs/ppt/hus/HUS2004Chartbk.ppt#16.

5. L. Cordain and others, "Origins and Evolution of the Western Diet: Health Implications for the 21st Century," *American Journal of Clinical Nutrition,* (2005): 81(2):341–54. Review.

6. G. Taubes, "The Soft Science of Dietary Fat," *Science,* 291 (2001): 2536–2545.

7. USDA, The Food Guide Pyramid, http://www.usda.gov/cnpp/pyrabklt.pdf.

8. CDC, "Trends in Intake of Energy and Macronutrients—United States, 1971–2000" *Morbidity and Mortality Weekly Report* (Feb 6, 2004): 53(04):80–82, http://www.cdc.gov/mmwr/preview/mmwrhtml/mm5304a3.htm.

9. W. C. Willet, M.D., *Eat, Drink, and Be Healthy* (New York: Free Press, 2001).

10. 5aday.org, "Consumption Statistics, Fruit and Vegetable Intake in the U.S.," http://www.5aday.com/html/research/consumptionstats.php.

CHAPTER 4

1. J. F. Neel, "The 'Thrifty Genotype' in 1998," *Nutrition Review* (1999): 57(5): S2–S9.
2. NAASO, The Obesity Society, "Lack of Sleep Leads to Excess Weight," Nov 16, 2004, http://www.naaso.org/news/20041116.asp.
3. J. E. Brody, "One-Two Punch for Losing Pounds: Exercise and Careful Diet," *The New York Times* on the Web, Oct 17, 2000, http://www.nytimes.com/2000/10/17 /science/17EXER.html?ex=1134968400&en=e61ba5491d27db2c&ei=5070.

CHAPTER 5

1. S. H. Holt and others, "A Satiety Index of Common Foods," *European Journal of Clinical Nutrition* (1995): 49(9):675–90.
2. D. S. Weigle and others, "A High-Protein Diet Induces Sustained Reductions in Appetite, Ad Libitum Caloric Intake, and Body Weight Despite Compensatory Changes in Diurnal Plasma Leptin and Ghrelin Concentrations," *American Journal of Clinical Nutrition* (2005): 82(1):41–8.
3. K. R. Westerterp, "Diet Induced Thermogenesis," *Nutrition & Metabolism* (2004): 1:5.
4. F. B. Hu and others, "Frequent Nut Consumption and Risk of Coronary Heart Disease in Women," *British Medical Journal* (Nov 14, 1998): 317:1341–5.
5. A. Ascherio and others, Harvard School of Public Health, "Trans Fatty Acids and Coronary Heart Disease," 1999, http://www.hsph.harvard.edu/reviews/transfats .html.
6. J. Brand-Miller, Low-Glycemic Index Diets in the Management of Diabetes: A Meta-Analysis of Randomized Controlled Trials," *Diabetes Care*, (2003): 26(8):2261–7.
7. K. Oh and others, "Carbohydrate Intake, Glycemic Index, Glycemic Load, and Dietary Fiber in Relation to Risk of Stroke in Women," *American Journal of Epidemiology*, (2005): 161(2):161–9.

CHAPTER 6

1. H. R. Farshchi and others, "Deleterious Effects of Omitting Breakfast on Insulin Sensitivity and Fasting Lipid Profiles in Healthy Lean Women," *American Journal of Clinical Nutrition* (2005): 81(2):388–96.
2. C. S. Johnson, "Strategies for Healthy Weight Loss: From Vitamin C to the Glycemic Response," *Journal of American College of Nutrition*, (2005): 24(3):158–65.
3. M. Boschmann and others, "Water-Induced Thermogenesis," *Journal of Clinical Endocrinology and Metabolism*, (2003): 88(12):6015–9.
4. E. Holmgren, "Myths & Facts: Alcohol and Weight," *Wines & Vines* (2004): http://www.findarticles.com/p/articles/mi_m3488/is_11_85/ai_n8576730.
5. Eureka Alert, "Coffee Is Number One Source of Antioxidants," (2005): http://search.eurekalert.org/e3/query.html?col=ev3rel&qc=ev3rel&op0=%2B&fl0=&ty 0=w&op1=%2B&fl1=keywords%3A&ty1=w&tx1=Medicine%2FHealth&tx0=coffee.
6. L. R. Young and others, "The Contribution of Expanding Portion Sizes to the U.S. Obesity Epidemic," *American Journal of Public Health*, (2002): 92:246–249.

CHAPTER 7

1. M. Chandalia and others, "Beneficial Effects of High Dietary Fiber Intake in Patients

with Type 2 Diabetes Mellitus," *New England Journal of Medicine* (2000) 342 (19):1392–1398.

2. NAASO, The Obesity Society, "Lack of Sleep Leads to Excess Weight," 2004, http://www.naaso.org/news/20041116.asp.

3. Science Daily, "Comfort-Food Cravings May Be Body's Attempt to Put Brake on Chronic Stress," Sept 6, 2006, http://www.sciencedaily.com/releases/ 2000/09 /000904122756.htm.

CHAPTER 8

1. T. A. Mori and others, "Effect of Fish Diets and Weight Loss on Serum Leptin Concentration in Overweight, Treated-Hypertensive Subjects. *Journal of Hypertension*, (2004): 22(10):1983–90.

2. M. Bhryn and others, "Omega-3 PUFA of Marine Origin Limit Diet-Induced Obesity in Mice by Reducing Cellularity of Adipose Tissue," *Lipids* (2004): 39:1177–1185.

3. M. S. Westerterp-Plantenga and others, "Sensory and Gastrointestinal Satiety Effects of Capsaicin on Food Intake," *International Journal of Obesity*, London (2005): 29(6):682–8.

4. M. Boschmann and others, "Water-Induced Thermogenesis," *Journal of Clinical Endocrinology and Metabolism* (2003): 88(12):6015–9.

5. M. S. Westerterp-Plantenga and others, Body Weight Loss and Weight Maintenance in Relation to Habitual Caffeine Intake and Green Tea Supplementation," *Obesity Research* (2005): 13(7):1195–204.

6. M. B. Zemel, "Role of Calcium and Dairy Products in Energy Partitioning and Weight Management," *American Journal of Clinical Nutrition* (2004): 79(5):907S–912S. Review.

CHAPTER 9

1. Food and Drug Administration (FDA), Center for Drug Evaluation, "FDA Announces Withdrawal Fenfluramine and Dexfenfluramine (Fen-Phen)," Sept 15, 1997, http://www.fda.gov/cder/news/phen/fenphenpr81597.htm.

2. ———, "Phenylpropanolamine & Risk of Hemorrhagic Stroke: Final Report of the Hemorrhagic Stroke Project," May 10, 2000, http://www.fda.gov/ohrms/dock ets/ac/00/backgrd/3647b1_tab19.doc.

3. United States Department of Agriculture, "What We Eat in America, NHANES 2000–2001: Usual Nutrient Intake from Food Compared to Dietary Reference Intakes," 2005, http://www.ars.usda.gov/SP2UserFiles/Place/12355000/pdf/usual intaketables2001–02.pdf.

4. C. S. Johnston, "Strategies for Healthy Weight Loss: From Vitamin C to the Glycemic Response, *Journal of American College or Nutrition* (2005): 24(3):158–65.

5. W. J. Evans, "Vitamin E, Vitamin C, and Exercise," *American Journal of Clinical Nutrition* (2000): 72(2 Suppl):647S–52S.

6. H. G. Preuss and others, "Citrusw Aurantium as a Thermogenic, Weight-Reduction Replacement for Ephedra: An Overview," *Journal of Medicine* (2002): 33(1–4):247–64.

7. A. Astrup and others, "The Effect and Safety of an Ephedrine/Caffeine Compound Compared to Ephedrine, Caffeine and Placebo in Obese Subjects on

an Energy Restricted Diet," *International Journal of Obesity Related Metabolism Disorders* (1992): 16(4):269–77.

8. S. Berude-Patrent and others, "Effects of Encapsulated Green Tea and Guarana Extracts Containing a Mixture of Epigallocatechin-3-Gallate and Caffeine on 24 Hour Energy Expenditure and Fat Oxidation in Men," *British Journal of Nutrition* (2005): 94(3):432–6.

9. J. M. Gaullier and others, "Conjugated Linoleic Acid Supplementation for 1 Year Reduces Body Fat Mass in Healthy Overweight Humans," *American Journal of Clinical Nutrition* (2004): 79(6):1118–25.

10. M. A. Belury and others, "The Conjugated Linoleic Acid (CLA) Isomer, t10c12-CLA, Is Inversely Associated with Changes in Body Weight and Serum Leptin in Subjects with Type 2 Diabetes Mellitus," *Journal Nutrition* (2003): 133(1):257S–260S. Review.

11. D. T. Villareal and others, "Effect of DHEA on Abdominal Fat and Insulin Action in Elderly Women and Men," *Journal of American Medical Association* (2004): 292(18):2243–2248.

12. D. E. Walsh and others, "Effect of Glucomannan on Obese Patients: a Clinical Study," *International Journal of Obesity* (1984): 8:289–93.

13. M. H. Pittler and others, Dietary Supplements for Body-Weight Reduction: A Systematic Review, *American Journal of Clinical Nutrition* (2004): 79(4):529–36. Review.

14. M. S. Kim and others, "Anti-Obesity Effects of Alpha-Lipoic Acid by Suppression of Hypothalamic AMP-Activated Protein Kinase," *Nature Medicine* (2004): 10(7):727–33. Epub 2004 Jun 13.

CHAPTER 10

1. M. A. Fiatarone and others, "Exercise Training and Nutritional Supplementation for Physical Frailty in Very Elderly People," *New England Journal of Medicine*, (1994): 330(25):1770–1775.

2. A. L. Dunn and others, "Comparison of Lifestyle and Structured Interventions to Increase Physical Activity and Cardiorespiratory Fitness. *Journal of American Medical Association* (1999): 281(4):327–34.

CHAPTER 13

1. FDA, "Mercury Levels in Commercial Fish and Shellfish," FDA Surveys 1990–2003, http://www.cfsan.fda.gov/~frf/sea-mehg.html.

INDEX

A

accountability, 11–12, 14, 107–108, 111, 121–123
aerobic exercise, 42–43, 84, 109–110
aging, 37–38
alcohol, 47, 67, 87–88, 133
alpha lipoic acid, 103
American Cancer Society, 8
American Journal of Clinical Nutrition, 23
American Sleep Apnea Association, 80
anaerobic/resistance exercise, 17, 84–85, 110–111, 117–119
antidepressants, 92
Antioxidant Research Laboratory of Tufts University, 93
antioxidants, 55, 68, 93, 98, 103
appetite
    and apple cider vinegar, 63
    and carbohydrates, 29, 44, 76
    controlling, 75–82
    drinks to control, 78–79
    emotional triggers, 80–81
    fiber to reduce, 76–77
    hunger, 1, 2–3, 29, 44, 46, 75–76, 81–82, 83
    hunger center in brain, 75–76, 102, 104
    and insulin, 27
    and portion sizes, 43–44
    and protein, 76
    and sleep, 79–80
    snacks to control, 77
    supplements to help control, 4, 81–82, 99
apple cider vinegar, 63
arthritis, 8
artificial sweeteners, 68, 69, 89
aspartame, 69
asthma drugs, 95

B

basal metabolic rate (BMR), 40–41, 83, 85
basal temperature testing, 37
beans and legumes, 52
beef
    choosing, 138
    Mushroom Burger, 175
    Oriental Beef Salad, 172
behavior change, 10, 12–15, 18
beta blockers, 39

body mass index (BMI), 16–17
body types, 34
bread, avoidance of, 64, 129
breakfast
    Beachcomber Tofu Scramble, 165
    best foods for, 61–62, 125–127
    eggs, 61–62, 126, 159–164
    foods to avoid, 128
    Green Eggs and Ham, 164
    Ham & Cheese Omelet, 161
    importance of, 60–61
    meal replacement, 62, 127–128
    Mini Breakfast Quiches, 160
    OC Scramble, 159
    Omelet Florentine, 163
    Tex-Mex Eggs, 162
    vegan options, 127

C

caffeine, 67–68, 78–79, 88–89, 95–96
calcium, 89–90
calories
    burning, 42–43, 46–47, 83–84
    increase in American consumption, 25–26
cancer, 8, 100
canned vegetables, 141
canola oil, 53
capsaicin, 86
carbohydrates
    avoidance of, 85–86
    caveman diet and, 22
    digestion of, 46–47
    excess, and obesity, 29–32
    fiber-rich, 55
    forms of, 27
    glycemic index (GI) of, 56–57
    glycemic load (GL) of, 58–59
    high-carbohydrate movement, 24–26
    high-glycemic, 29, 48
    and hunger, 29, 44, 76
    and insulin, 27–28, 29
    and low-fat diets, 3
    modern consumption of, 23–27
    from refined grains, 55
    simple vs. complex, 28
    supplements to cut cravings, 81–82, 99